The English Medieval Hospital

The English Medieval Hospital
Hospital
c. 1050-1640

Elizabeth Prescott

Seaby

Elizabeth Prescott 1992
First published 1992
Photoset by Setrite

Printed and bound by
The Cromwell Press Limited,
Broughton Gifford, Melksham,
Wiltshire

ISBN 1 85264 054 5

A CIP Catalogue record
for this book is available
from the British Library.

CONTENTS

ACKNOWLEDGEMENTS

The author and publisher wish to thank the following for permission to use the following photographs: Royal Commission on the Historical Monuments of England, 2, 4, 6, 8, 10, 11, 12, 14, 15, 17, 18, 19, 20, 21, 22, 23, 25, 26, 28, 31, 33, 36, 43, 44, 45, 46, 47, 48, 50, 51, 55, 58, 60, 61; BT Batsford Ltd, 1, 5, 24, 30, 35, 37, 38, 39, 40, 41, 52, 53, 56, 57, 59, 62, 63; English Heritage, 9; County Life, 13; Courtauld Institute, 27; Times Newspapers, 49

PREFACE

Few people realize that there were almost as many medieval hospitals and almshouse foundations in England as there were the more well-known monasteries. Many were lost alongside the monasteries in the Reformation and yet none were converted like the monasteries at, for example, Titchfield and Netley into gracious private homes or have been so well preserved as ruins as at Fountains or Rievaulx. So what were these hospitals, what were they like and what did they do?

Surprisingly perhaps, several of these medieval hospitals are still fulfilling their original function today. Rarely have the buildings survived almost intact as they do at St Mary's Chichester, St Cross, Winchester or Ford's Coventry, painstakingly rebuilt after being bombed during the Second World War but each fragment, archway or chapel contributes to the story. It is a story of continuous evolution of both function and design readily identifiable today in the wards of the large hospitals or in the tranquillity of the modern almshouse complex.

Any age reveals much of itself in its architecture. The major buildings of medieval England; the abbeys and priories, castles, churches and cathedrals and the larger houses are well known, the hospitals and almshouses much less so. Sir Nicholas Pevsner's *The Buildings of England* series were invaluable for identification of surviving building and the files of the National Almshouse Association were of great assistance in verifying the continued existence of some sites, particularly those of post-Reformation date. In all, over 200 sites were identified as having standing remains and came into existence between *c.* 1050 and 1640. Hospitals which were monastic infirmaries or which never enjoyed an independent existence have not been included; neither have those institutions which belonged to the military orders.

This book seeks to highlight the changes and development of the medieval hospital and almshouses as seen through their architecture. The buildings are a particularly rich source of information when there is a paucity of primary source material. Few hospital accounts have survived — some foundations had already lost their records by the Dissolution and many have perished since. The more secular nature and increasing number of non-religious foundations since 1350 also reduced the chances of survival.

The records of the local historical and archaeological societies have
been particularly useful in tracing the history of individual sites but there
have been few attempts to examine hospitals and almshouses on a country-
wide scale. Many studies provide a valuable insight into the internal organization of hospitals but contain little information on changes to the fabric.
Furthermore studies generally cease at the Reformation whereas many
hospitals survived, prospered and developed their eelimosinary role.

In recent years there have been attempts, most notable at Ospringe and
Canterbury in Kent to use both archaeological and historical data to trace
developments at individual sites. The last decade has also seen a notable
increase in the number of books and articles on aspects of the history of
medicine and excavations such as at St Giles Hospital, Brompton Bridge,
North Yorkshire reveal a growing interest in this neglected area of study.
It is hoped that this book will emphasize the importance of the medieval
hospital and almshouse and gain them a recognized significance in the
medieval scene.

CHAPTER ONE

INTRODUCTION

The earliest hospitals were founded in Saxon times although few of that age can be dated with any certainty. A great many more were founded in the eleventh and twelfth centuries, and by the end of the thirteenth century over 500 hospitals had been established in England alone. The rate of growth slowed down after the Black Death but by 1547 between 700 and 800 foundations were in existence. A considerable proportion of these earlier foundations were lost at the Dissolution. However, from *c.* 1550 a new impetus for foundation created many hundreds more. By 1642 this movement was forced to draw to a close with the beginning of the Civil War. A complete series of buildings representing foundations from most of these dates persists to the present and provides examples of the architecture and plans successively in use. Although closely allied to the monks and monastic tradition, this book seeks to place in context those buildings which can be distinguished, by archaeological and documentary records, as having an existence independent of their monastic counterparts.

Like the monasteries, the medieval hospitals were a mixture of the aesthetic and the functional and there were many changes to their plan and design throughout their history. It is the purpose of this book to chart these alterations and place them in their social and historical context.

The medieval hospital, unlike the modern institution, was not a building specifically for the cure of the body. Medieval hospitals fulfilled a wide range of obligations, sometimes as a specialized unit or, more often, discharging several functions. From early times the provision of hospitality for travellers, in keeping with monastic traditions, gave rise to the institution known as the *Maison Dieu, Domus Dei* or God's House. This class of hospital became particularly numerous in the decades of the great period of pilgrimage in England following the murder of Thomas à Becket in 1170 with the foundation of several houses in the southern ports − Dover, Portsmouth, Southampton and along the main routes to London. Hospitals were also built at other popular centres of pilgrimage − Walsingham, Durham and Glastonbury. This function continued to be significant in the larger cities, ports and major trade routes throughout the Middle Ages. In 1464 St Bartholomew's Hospital in London was still offering relief to travellers, being granted pardon by the king for obtaining unauthorized grants because of the relief given there to 'poor pilgrims, soldiers, sailors and others of all nations' (*CPR 1461-67*: 323). The giving of hospitality leaves no permanent trace in the buildings of hospitals. Smaller hospitals, such as at Chapel Plaster, may have existed solely for this purpose. More often it was performed as a charitable duty, its importance underlined by the continuance of the ancient custom of giving bread and ale to all travellers which can still be found at the gate of St Cross Hospital, Winchester.

Situated on the major route between Southampton and Winchester, St Cross Hospital must have been much in demand for hospitality. Nevertheless it was only a minor function of the hospital. Another minor function carried out at St Cross Hospital, and at several others too, was the offering of some form of charitable education. In the mid-fifteenth century, seven choristers were educated at St Cross Hospital; in 1259 twelve scholars were supported at St Mark's Hospital, Bristol and the London hospitals of St Anthony and St Bartholomew became so noted for the high standards of education meted to the poor and orphaned children that they started to attract fee-paying pupils (for the hospitals of London, *see* Rawcliffe 1984). Again, the fulfilling of this function leaves little impact on the design or architecture of the buildings.

Neither were hospitals designed with any specific medical facilities. Many of the early hospitals were administered by religious brethren or sisters and either followed, or were influenced by, the Augustinian rule. This particular rule laid emphasis on the need for involvement in society, and, with spiritual duties lighter than those of other monastic orders, left more time for the care of the sick. However, salvation of the body was unimportant and almost certainly beyond the competence of the carers. From the early thirteenth century, Christian dogma forbade surgical incision or any other treatment which involved the shedding of blood, and where sickness was still connected with sin, healing began with prayer and penance.

Nevertheless some doctors did attend the hospitals. Before the Black Death there are records of only five doctors who were connected in any way with hospitals. Between 1349 and 1530 the records show fifty doctors associated with hospitals, all physicians or surgeons (Gottfried 1986: 260). Provision was also made for barbers, as at St Nicholas Hospital, Salisbury, in 1478. These barbers, of whom the records increase in the later Middle Ages, may have been associated with the barber-surgeons, members of the larger company of barbers and rivals to the surgeons. Perhaps attendance of a doctor in some form or other was more common than generally realized, although patients probably had a better chance of becoming well if left alone. At best, the medicine offered by medieval physicians was based on a theoretical mixture of the rational and magic. The physicians were the social élite of medical doctors but medicine was still only a minor subject at the English universities and Christian theory prevented the development of practice and study of anatomy and physiology. It was only through the opportunities granted by the wars of the fourteenth and fifteenth centuries, and the development of printing, that the surgeons began to make advances in their craft. Most of the changes in late medieval medicine were in surgery rather than physic, yet the development of medicine as a whole foundered in the wake of the strict medical hierarchy.

Salvation of the body was unimportant. A far greater influence on the design and layout of the pre-Reformation medieval hospital building was in carrying out its primary function – the salvation and remembrance of souls. It was strongly believed that the sick and poor should spend their time in hospital in pursuit of a communal life to pray for the souls of others. The most active period of hospital foundation took place when the concept of purgatory was widely accepted and the efficacy of prayers for the dead to hasten passage made charitable giving rich in rewards for benefactors and founders. The founding of a hospital provided the intercessionary prayers of the living in pursuit of spiritual salvation, but it also allowed the opportunity for an elaborate memorial to the generosity of the founder or benefactor.

Despite having a common purpose, the early hospitals were founded in widely differing circumstances; for many of them little is known of their early history and it is likely that most of the smaller hospitals have disappeared from the architectural or archaeological record. A hospital could be founded by anyone but they could not have a chapel or oratory attached without episcopal licence. It is the remains of the larger foundations in which mass was celebrated, confessions heard, burial and other parochial rights obtained, that give us clues to the organization, design and subsequent changes to the medieval hospital.

Other clues may be found in the siting of the hospitals. In the early Middle Ages, founders usually followed well-known conventions when choosing a site for their institution. The leper hospital, for example, was a small category of hospital with a clearly defined specialized function. Leprosy was widespread in the twelfth and thirteenth centuries and was considered not only physically contagious but also invoked fear of moral contamination. Strict rules were laid down regarding the conduct and organization of lepers. After a special church service, the unfortunate victim was enjoined never again to enter a church, market, mill, bakehouse or any other assembly of people. Furthermore, lepers were to wear a special dress so that other people could avoid contamination and, as an extra precaution, a leper was not permitted to wash his hands or belongings in any water that would be used by others. Thus leper foundations were nearly always sited outside the town boundaries and downstream from springs and rivers; examples are the lazar houses at Nottingham, Hereford, Cambridge, Canterbury and Southampton. St Giles Hospital, London, acquired its name 'in the fields' from being so far out in the countryside. The sites of leper hospitals can often be identified from the survival of their dedication, for example to St Mary Magdalene, or from the existence of a leper well. The disease began to die out in England in the fourteenth century and only twelve new foundations are known after 1350. However, lepers were never allowed to be fully professed into the religious discipline although they often lived a quasi-religious life, as at St Giles, Durham. It is likely that many smaller communities, living on alms, existed but they have left no trace in the architectural or documentary records.

The changing economic and social world of the later Middle Ages, with the erosion of the communal and spiritual life, was reflected in considerable changes in the plan and design of hospitals. From the mid-fourteenth century, the foundation, design and function of the medieval hospital began to change considerably. With the decline in monastic ideals and, in particular, decreasing emphasis on the communal life, the provision and maintenance of newly founded hospitals became increasingly the preserve of the laity. The smaller hospital or, as it more often became, the almshouse, formed the focus of charitable giving alongside the parish church, the friary and the chantry. Urban and rural communities alike attempted to meet the needs of the poor and infirm with the new smaller almshouses which were easier to administer and control. The foundation at Tattershall in 1485-6 is typical of the more substantial new foundation of its time. In fulfilment of the wishes of the founder, it was built as part of a collegiate establishment, adjoining the churchyard, with a common hall and chapel, and thirteen separate chambers for the bedesmen's use. The bedesmen were being supported, yet living within a college still provided for the salvation of the soul of the founder.

As the focus on the communal and even spiritual buildings declined, improvements to the living conditions of the hospital inmates continued. Private rooms and other comforts provided for the occupants forced changes to the layout of the new foundations and alterations to the older establishments. These changes resulted in a marked difference of hospital plan and design which can be seen taking place from the thirteenth through to the seventeenth century.

The developments in hospital design, moving towards smaller, more comfortable establishments with the emphasis on privacy, should not be viewed in isolation. Rising standards and expectations were characteristic of late medieval society and they affected contemporary life outside the hospital as well as inside it. Thus the private chambers of the hospitals and almshouses have their equivalent in the partitioned and divided dormitories and refectories of the religious houses.[1] Improved lodgings for hospital masters and wardens are matched by rebuilt abbots' quarters.[2] In each of these places, advances in heating and sanitation, with glazing and framed staircases to follow, have become recognizable as standard features,[3] also to be seen in the castles and manor-houses, the rectories, vicarages and chantry houses, the burgess and yeoman dwellings of the period. The hospital, as may be expected, was part of the changing scene; these changes and developments can be clearly seen in the hospitals and almshouses featured in this book.

CHAPTER TWO

THE EARLY HOSPITALS
c. 1200-1350

The earliest surviving hospital architecture dates from the twelfth century. It is probable at this time that, in common with other important domestic and ecclesiastical architecture, stone structures replaced some of the original wooden buildings of the earliest foundations. The large new twelfth-century hospitals, as indicated by their standing remains or revealed by excavation, were likely to have been built in stone from the first. The plans of these remains indicate a basic standard design for their construction tempered by local variations.

The organization and layout of the hospital were largely determined by the need to provide for the bodily needs of the inmates and more especially for the care of their souls. Characteristic of these early hospitals was the arrangement whereby the inmates were accommodated under one roof with a chapel adjoining – this plan is known as the 'infirmary-hall' type. The hall might vary in length, for example from only four bays at the hospital of St John the Baptist, High Wycombe, founded in 1117, to sixteen bays at the Newarke Hospital, Leicester, founded in 1331. The foundation of the Newarke Hospital virtually marked the last of the buildings of this type.

One group of buildings which did not conform to the standard plan were the early leper hospitals. Lepers were barred, or removed, from the almshouses and hospitals once they contracted the disease. The lazar houses probably differed in their arrangement, in order to cater for the conditions imposed upon the lepers by the peculiarities of their disease. Isolation was insisted upon in early times and was achieved, as at the hospital of St John the Baptist, Harbledown, by groups of individual cottages set in an enclosure with a chapel and a well. (Leper wells also survive at Winchester and Lyme Regis.) From the later thirteenth century the evidence suggests that lepers were accommodated, at least in the larger hospitals, in buildings which followed a more standard plan, such as that to be found at the foundation of St Martha and St Lazarus at Sherburn.

But frequently leper hospitals were extremely small, perhaps providing accommodation for only two or three inmates. As with the other smaller hospitals, many have disappeared leaving little or no trace of their layout. A rare example of a small hospital survives at Chapel Plaster. This hospital probably provided a refuge for travellers and pilgrims visiting nearby Glastonbury. The surviving remains date from the late fourteenth century, but the hospital was probably built much earlier and subsequently altered, as it was again in the next century. Chapel Plaster represents a typical example of a small foundation which grew or changed on an *ad hoc* basic with no discernible standard plan.

The hospital complex

Many of these early hospitals were founded at the same time as the great twelfth-century boom in monastic building. Like the monasteries, the early hospitals sometimes had to fulfil the needs of quite large communities. As well as providing for the inmates, the foundations supported considerable numbers of staff. In 1135 St Cross Hospital near Winchester maintained four chaplains, thirteen clerks, seven choristers, a master and a steward. At the same date, the hospital of St Giles, Kepier, Durham, supported thirteen brethren who performed duties familiar to those of a large monastic estate. For both inmates and brethren a large number and variety of buildings were required, probably much akin to those provided for a typical monastic complex.

The meagre archaeological evidence surviving from St Giles, Durham, is suggestive of precisely such a complex (*see* Parsons 1968). But remains of domestic buildings of the early hospitals are scarce and few investigations have extended beyond the hall and chapel. Recent excavations over a considerable area of the precinct of the hospital of St Mary at Ospringe, founded in the early thirteenth century, reveal important evidence as to the nature of the early hospital complex. The hospital at Ospringe was situated on both sides of Watling Street, with the main complex lying to the north. Excavations revealed buildings which formed part of a neatly laid out precinct (Smith 1979; Drake 1914), probably surrounded by a wall, with the infirmary hall and chapel providing the pivot around which the rest of the hospital buildings were constructed. At the north end of the hall a single-storeyed building constructed of flint was revealed, probably eight bays in length, with a central arcade of stone pillars. To the north of it was situated, as on many monastic sites, the reredorter, served by a stone-lined culvert which ran under the floor of the hall. The chapel adjoined the hall in the centre of its eastern side and at right angles to it. A clear division of function was identified between the buildings on either side of the culvert. To the west was the infirmary hall, reredorter and all the domestic buildings including the kitchen, service yard with pond, bakehouse, brewhouse and also the cemetery. To the east lay the chapel and gatehouse (known from documentary evidence) and a small close of buildings sited to the north-east of the infirmary hall.

The domestic buildings to the east of the culvert at Ospringe are strikingly similar to those associated with a self-supporting monastic community. Evidence elsewhere supports this comparability. The brethren of many of these foundations lived as the religious. A typical example is the hospital of St John the Baptist, Bedford, founded *c.* 1180, where the brethren had a common dormitory and refectory. The brethren of this hospital followed the rule of St Augustine, taking an oath of obedience to the statutes and the master. They had the tonsure of a priest and wore clothing of any suitable colour covered by a dark mantle. They were to remain in the hospital for life and were, every day, to sing the canonical hours and celebrate divine office for the living and the dead, praying especially for the soul of the founder and other benefactors.

Like the hospital of St John the Baptist, Bedford, many of the other early hospital foundations followed or were much influenced by monastic rule. Most commonly it was that of the Augustinian order since that particular order was one of the few able to accommodate the secular needs of the hospital. The hospital of St John the Baptist, Bedford, adapted the rule of St Augustine to their particular circumstances when, in 1306, Bishop Dalderby referred to the three rules of obedience, chastity and poverty 'but above all things charity' (*VCH Bedfordshire 3*: 397). They were, unusually, allowed to speak in soft tones in the refectory, although the usual strict silence was enforced in the church, cloister and dormitory. These adaptations of the rules suggest that the hospitals, despite their similarities in plan to the monastic institutions, were more open and secular in nature than were their monastic counterparts. This is well illustrated at St Mary's Hospital, Ospringe. There is no doubt that the only standing remains on the site are the stone walls of two undercrofts, dating to *c.* 1255 and *c.* 1300, which are situated outside the main hospital precinct and separated from it by Watling Street. These undercrofts were built to carry either first-floor halls or the solars of ground-floors halls and, as such, probably formed the residences of the permanent brethren. Thus the staff quarters were situated in a much more open position. The brethren at Ospringe were known as *presbyteri conversi* or 'secular priests'. These priests were supported by two secular clerks and would not have been subject to the same restrictions as the monastic brethren in the enclosed orders. This more open arrangement is further supported by the existence of private apartments for secular use within the main precinct of the hospital.

The infirmary hall: the plan

Thus the hospital complex was very similar to the monastic precinct. The design of the infirmary hall itself must also have owed its origins to monastic precedents as, for example, at the eleventh-century infirmary of Canterbury Cathedral Priory (1). Here extant remains and the results of excavation reveal the basic plan for the earliest hospitals. Characteristically, it consisted of a long hall, narrow in relation to its length, with or without

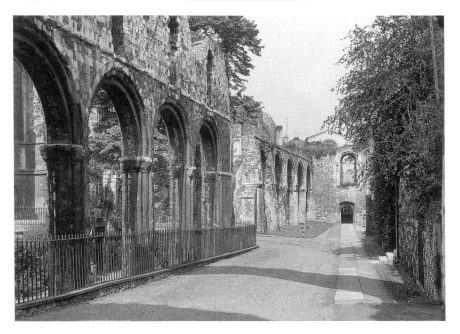

1   Monastic precedents, like the eleventh-century infirmary hall of Canterbury Cathedral Priory, may have influenced the design of the early hospitals.

aisles, terminating in or adjoined by a chapel. The attached chapel had the special feature of allowing direct communication to the hall. The infirmary hall with its chapel are frequently referred to as 'nave and chancel' respectively on account of their similarity in plan to those parts of a church.

Indeed, the hospital of St Thomas of Canterbury at Ramsey (2), founded *c.* 1180, needed little alteration when the hospital became a parish church in the mid-thirteenth century. A south chapel was added, and a tower, a feature not normally associated with the earliest hospitals, was built on to the westernmost bay of the nave. The arcades of the late-twelfth-century building, which consisted of an infirmary hall of eight bays with north and south aisles, each 4 m in width, are original. Adjoining the hall was the main chapel and, in addition, there were north and south chapels which would have extended across and served the north and south aisles. Thus the interior gives a very good impression of the infirmary-hall type of hospital in its early years clearly showing the importance of the link between hall and chapel.

The best surviving example of a hospital of the infirmary-hall type is St Mary's at Chichester, founded *c.* 1158 (3) but constructed on its present site between *c.* 1290 and 1300. The entrance to the infirmary hall was through an archway and passage which formed the western end of the hall. Although the two western bays of the hall are no longer in existence,

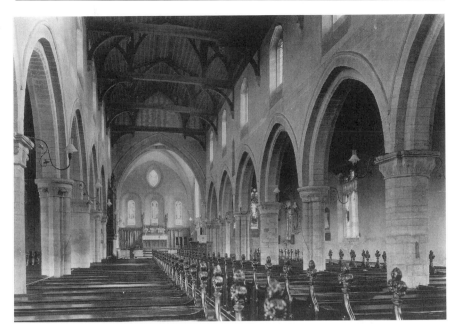

2 The hospital of St Thomas of Canterbury, Ramsey, easily converted into a parish church in the mid-thirteenth century.

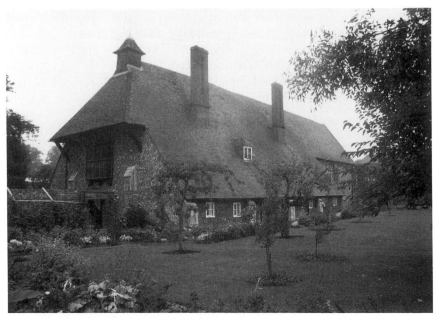

3 St Mary's, Chichester, one of the best surviving examples of the twelfth-century infirmary-hall hospital.

it originally comprised six bays forming a total length of 36.6 m. The width throughout was 13.7 m, making for a spacious hall divided into a central area and aisles by wooden pillars. These pillars support the massive and splendid timber roof which continues to within 1.8 m of the ground, resting on low stone walls pierced by small windows under which the beds of the inmates would have been placed. The chapel occupies only 6.7 m of the eastern end of the hall and is separated from it by a rich screen, a common arrangement for the division of hall and chapel. Since recourse to prayer was frequent, this arrangement afforded an opportunity for the inmates to be in close proximity to the altar, a provision especially important for the sick unable to leave their beds.

The infirmary-hall plans seen at Ramsey, Chichester and also found at Northampton (*c.* 1140), Canterbury (*c.* 1133), High Wycombe (*c.* 1180) and elsewhere (St John the Baptist, Huntingdon, 1170-90; St Giles, Norwich, 1246; God's House, Portsmouth, *c.* 1212), undoubtedly represent the most common early hospital design. But there were several important variations on this arrangement. The simplest of these was a straightforward aisleless hall with attached chapel in the same range, as seen at the hospital of St Katherine at Ledbury, founded in 1232 and already rebuilt on the same site in *c.* 1330-40. At Ledbury the total length of the range is 28.3 m of which, as at Chichester, no more than 6.7 m were assigned to the chapel. The width throughout the hall was 9.1 m, the only division betwen the separate parts of the building being a simple timber truss.

A more elaborate variation of the plan is represented at the hospital of St Thomas the Martyr at Canterbury, founded soon after Archbishop Becket's murder in 1170. Here the infirmary hall, originally of five bays, was supplied with a western aisle. But more exceptional at Canterbury — and here it differed from Chichester, Ramsey or Ledbury — was the hospital's two-storeyed construction, the first-floor hall being set over a substantial vaulted undercroft of identical plan, clearly datable to about 1180 (4).

St Thomas's may have served as the model for the two-storeyed infirmary hall with terminating chapel seen also at St Mary's Hospital, Dover, shortly before 1221. These two hospitals also share an unusual characteristic: the chapel is set at right angles to the infirmary hall and in the centre of one side. This feature has already been observed at St Mary's Hospital, Ospringe, and it is also found in an interesting group of other Kentish foundations, either earlier or contemporary: St John the Baptist, Canterbury, of the late eleventh century; St Mary's Strood, founded *c.* 1192-3. Of this modification to the design — only to be found in the early Kent hospitals — only St Bartholomew's, Chatham (1077-1108) differs. Here the chapel is situated at one end of the building. This may be explained by the need to accommodate the buildings on a restricted site.

Of this early Kentish group the hospital of St John the Baptist, Canterbury, illustrates yet another interesting variation of the infirmary-hall type of

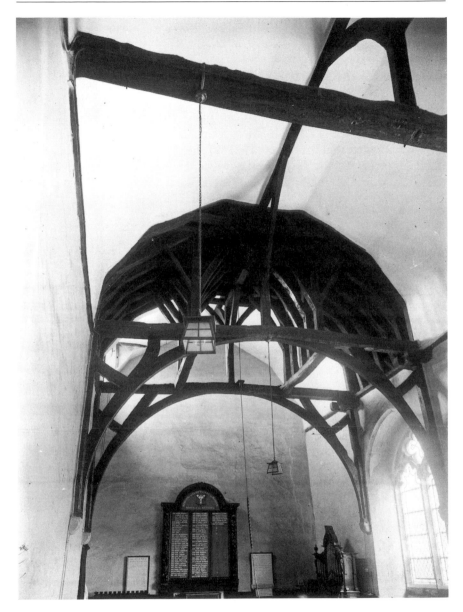

4   The chapel of St Thomas the Martyr, Canterbury, set at right-angles to the hall, a feature only to be found in Kent.

plan. The right-angled chapel, as well as the infirmary hall, were divided across the width into two halves, enabling each section of the hall to communicate with its individual chapel. Eadmer writes that Lanfranc, when Archbishop of Canterbury, built a 'decent and ample house of stone' outside the north gate of the city for the benefit of poor and infirm persons and divided it into two parts for men and women (Clay 1909: 106). Lanfranc's endowment was for the maintenance of thirty persons of each sex, and the design of his hospital well suited the segregation of the sexes.

St Nicholas's Hospital, Salisbury, solved the problem of segregation of the sexes in a different manner. Founded shortly before 1227, the hospital was soon rebuilt on a new site a little to the south, probably in 1231 when royal grants were made of timber 'for building the hospital' (*CClR 1231-2*: 14-15). The new foundation consisted of a single-storeyed infirmary hall, 36.6 × 15.2 m, divided down the centre by an arcade of seven arches. This formed two separate aisles, each with its own pitched roof and each terminated by a chapel at the east and a porch on the west. This obligation to care for the sick and poor of both sexes is reflected in another way at Lewes, Sussex. In an early deed the parish is described as that of St John the Baptist and St Mary Magdalen, two common dedications of the early hospitals. It is likely that here, too, the hospital was divided into two wards for men and women, each with its appropriately dedicated altar at the east end. Other hospitals with a similar double dedication no doubt also served this purpose.

All the above examples of the infirmary-hall type of foundation were purpose-built to serve as hospitals. In some instances a private dwelling was adapted for use as a hospital. When this occurred, the evidence suggests that they were, nevertheless, concerned to maintain the basic design, converting the building into the standard plan of hall with terminating chapel, as far as space would allow, with adaptations and improvements carried out to fit the model as funds permitted. The best documented example, also investigated by excavation, is the hospital of St Mary, Canterbury. The hospital was founded by Alexander of Gloucester *c.* 1200 but the first building known on the site was a stone house rebuilt by Lambin Frese, a moneyer, in 1180. The foundations and all the lower parts of the north and south walls of the present building may date back to *c.* 1175 but the founding of the hospital initiated a major phase of reconstruction. To form the chapel, the porch of Frese's house was demolished and the chapel constructed, significantly, in common with other early foundations in Kent, at right angles to the existing range, although the restricted nature of the site probably prevented it from being placed in the centre of one side. A new wall was constructed, continuing the east frontage wall of the chapel and forming a room to the north-west, probably used as a kitchen for it retains a late-twelfth-century fireplace. The hall was constructed over the original house some time in the thirteenth century, a new floor being laid and benches built on the south-west and north-west sides of the rooms. Documentary evidence suggests that these fine buildings were in a ruinous condition by the mid-fourteenth century and the hospital was extensively rebuilt in the late fourteenth century on the same site but with certain modifications to the interior (Detsicas 1981).

The strength of the tradition of the infirmary-hall plan is well illustrated even in the small, short-lived foundation of St Nicholas and St Katherine of Canterbury. The hospital was founded shortly before 1203 by William Cockyn, a citizen of Canterbury, who had purchased the property adjoining his own in St Peter's Street. By the end of 1203 the foundation was united with the hospital of St Thomas the Martyr at Eastbridge but not before Cockyn had added an aisled infirmary hall, probably of two bays to the rear of the original building.

The dominant standard plan of infirmary hall with chapel is well observed at St Giles Hospital, Norwich, (5) which served both as a hospital and a parish church. The hospital was founded in 1249 by the Bishop of Norwich and erected on a prescribed plot of ground opposite the existing parish church of St Helen and under the walls of the priory. Soon after construction of the hospital, St Helen's church was demolished, provision having already been made within the hospital for the parish church by creating space between the long aisled infirmary hall and the aisleless chapel to the east. This space, in which was placed the parish altar of St Helen, formed an elaborately vaulted south 'transept' entered from the south by a separate long porch of three vaulted bays. Thus, St Helen's,

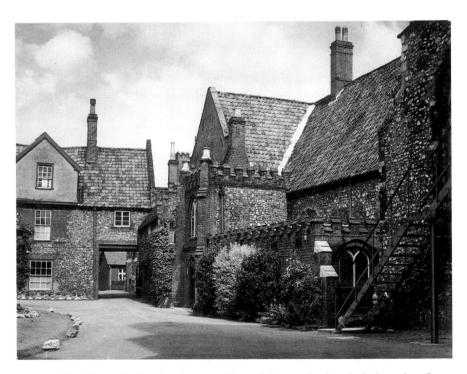

5 St Giles, Norwich, showing incorporation of the parish chapel, dedicated to St Helen, in the centre of the infirmary hall.

without being allowed to interfere with the normal arrangement of infirmary hall with terminating chapel, formed an integral part of the hospital, expanding the eastern end of the building and extending its overall length to just over 61 m (Bennett-Symons 1925).

The tradition of infirmary hall with attached chapel remained the standard method of hospital construction, and continued, at least for the larger foundations, until the early fourteenth century. Major reconstruction work such as took place at St Katherine's Hospital, Ledbury, was extremely rare. Where rebuilding did take place it was quite often necessitated by poor original siting. Such was the case at the hospital of St John the Baptist, Coventry, founded early in the reign of Henry II but situated at the foot of the northern slope of a valley close to two streams on a very low level. The hospital was subject to frequent flooding and the site was abandoned but had been rebuilt by the early fourteenth century on higher ground to the north. Significantly, like St Katherine's, Ledbury, the new infirmary hall of the Coventry hospital was also built to the standard design.

A different problem was faced by Bishop Glanville's foundation of St Mary at Strood: poor workmanship. The chapel collapsed in the later thirteenth century, less than 100 years after foundation, bringing down with it much of the infirmary hall. The right-angled chapel and infirmary hall, divided down the centre, much akin to St John's Hospital, Canterbury, was constructed anew but on the same ground plan; new material was laid on top of the stumps of the old walls and the new walls were built on top of this, making occasional use of the dressed and carved stone surviving from the earlier building. A new floor of plain tiles was laid on more than 30 cm of rubble from the old building. Once again the infirmary-hall plan was preferred.

St Mary's was a small foundation, continually in dispute with the monks of Rochester, and may never have been able to afford more than basic repairs. In contrast, St Leonard's Hospital, York, was refounded on a new site and enlarged in 1135 for the reception of poor people. The hospital was the largest institution of its kind in the country, consisting of a master, 13 brethren, 4 secular priests, 8 sisters, 30 choristers, 2 schoolmasters, 206 bedesmen and 6 servitors. It was richly endowed and yet in 1309, when the foundation was again increased, it merely enlarged the dwelling house, i.e. the infirmary hall (*CPR 1307-13*: 190).

Considerable expansion was carried out at St Mary's Hospital, Dover, in the early fourteenth century. A second infirmary hall, built to the standard design, with its own chapel, was added to the south of the original hall, separated from it by a stone arcade of considerable proportions. This second hall survives; an impressive sight when viewed from the south, with its six great four-light geometric windows with buttresses between them. St Mary's was a prestigious institution, founded *c.* 1220 for the maintenance of the poor and infirm as well as pilgrims, by Hugh de

Burgh, Earl of Kent and Justiciary of England, and was well supported, especially after the transfer of the patronage to Henry III who granted the hospital a large number of charters. St Mary's and St Leonard's undoubtedly would have built the finest they could afford. Yet both chose to build in the traditional manner — a tribute to the endurance of the infirmary-hall plan for over 200 years.

The infirmary hall: the interior

Evidence is scarce as to how these infirmary halls were furnished and decorated. Now and then the statutes give a rare glimpse of life in the halls. At St David's Hospital, Kingsthorpe, founded towards the end of the twelfth century, the statutes, laid down in some detail, reveal that 'in the body of the house adjoining the chapel of the Holy Trinity there should be three rows of beds joined together in length in which the poor and strangers and invalids may lie for the purpose of hearing mass and attending prayers more easily and conveniently' (Markham 1897-8: 170). In the earliest times these beds probably consisted of pallets of straw. But in 1294 at God's House Hospital, Southampton, a gift of five oaks was granted to repair the beds of the infirm and it is probable that wooden bedsteads had been introduced by the late twelfth century.

Within the hall at St David's, Kingsthorpe, there were two chapels, dedicated to the Holy Trinity and St David; one bell summoned the brethren and inmates to prayer. There would undoubtedly have been a lamp burning in the centre of the hall, if not by each bed, with bequests often granted to provide lighting, enabling the sick to look upon the altar at all times. Grants were also recorded for the necessary items of linen, blankets and clothing. A typical grant was made to St Bartholomew's Hospital, London, in 1215 when Alexander de Norfolk left a house to the hospital so that the revenues might be used to provide shelter for the poor and linen sheets for the infirmary. Whenever possible, however, inmates were expected to bring with them their own blankets which were retained in the event of their death. Dark robes, hoods or cloaks were worn by the brethren and also, apparently, the inmates, for the statutes of St David's reveal that the old garments of the brethren were 'conferred on the poor by the disposition of the master and brethren' (Markham 1897-8: 170).

Since many of the early hospital foundations provided for travellers, they would have needed to be 'furnished with beds and other necessaries for the entertainment of poor travellers' as at the hospital of St Anne and St Louis, Brentford (Clay 1909: 8). Other hospitals also offered total provision for the genuinely sick poor, as at St John the Baptist, Bedford, where 'all needy persons born of the town of Bedford, who had become poor by misfortune rather than by fault, might seek admittance and be maintained' (*VCH Bedfordshire* 3: 396). As both hospitals were places of temporary refuge, all the necessary food and clothing must have been provided by the foundation. This was most likely common practice and it was still followed by the Elsing Spital, London, in 1448 when an inventory, listing the contents of the buttery, kitchen, great and little chambers, library and treasury, revealed that blankets, beds and readers (*lectorum*) when worn out were to be replaced by the *custos* (warden). The inventory also discloses that the house, probably typical of its kind, had an income of £198 16s. 4d. but owed debts of £160 7s. 9d. (*VCH London* 1: 536). It is, therefore, likely that these institutions were somewhat sparsely furnished. Few inventories of contents survive to confirm the evidence, but one of 1303 from St Bartholomew's Hospital, Bristol, reveals the contents of the 'house', probably the refectory. The only items listed are three tables with trestles, three basins with three copper ewers and one damaged basin (*Trans. Bristol and Gloucester Arch. Soc.* 1958: 180).

If evidence for the furnishings of the halls is scarce then so, too, is the evidence for their decoration. However, what survives suggests that schemes of embellishment may, on occasion, have been quite lavish. At the hospital of St Thomas the Martyr, Canterbury, a fine late-twelfth-century wall-painting depicting a seated figure of Christ Blessing survives (**6**). This painting is situated on the hall side of the dividing wall between hall and chapel and may mark the position of a hall altar or be representative of a scheme of decoration of the infirmary hall similar to the wall-paintings of contemporary parish churches.

The chapel

> Wherefore, beloved brethren in the Lord, I deliver and commit to Providence and to the administration of yourselves and your successors (as evidenced by this writing) the Hospital of the poor of Christ, which I, for the health of my soul, and the souls of my predecessors, and of the Kings of England, have founded anew without the walls of Winchester ... (Dollman and Jobbins 1859-63, 1: 9).

So runs the mid-twelfth-century foundation charter of the hospital of St Cross, Winchester, attributable to Bishop Henry of Blois. St Cross was constituted to receive 100 other poor 'impotent' men referred to as the 'poor in Christ' who may 'there humbly and devotedly serve God' (Dollman and Jobbins 1859-63, 1: 9). Indeed, in the early hospitals care of the soul was considered to be of far greater importance than care of the body, and service to God was the ultimate concern of every member of the hospital community.

Of particular importance, as in any religious institution of the time, was the soul of the founder himself. For the sake of his soul, Henry of Blois began at St Cross the finest of all the surviving hospital chapels. In the absence of firm documentary evidence the architecture of St Cross has

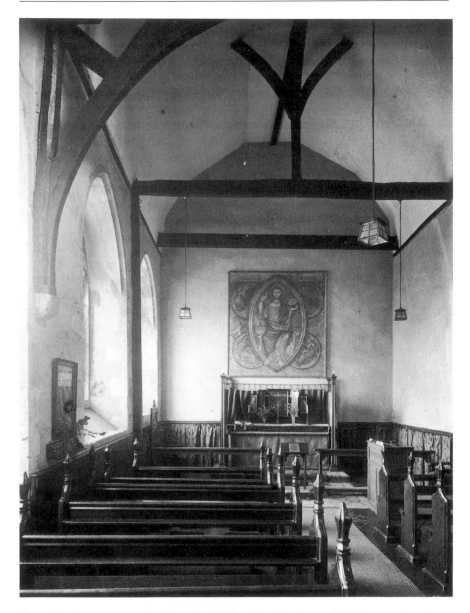

6   Twelfth-century wall-painting, in the hall of St Thomas the Martyr, Canterbury.

recently been intensively studied to reveal its history and development (a comprehensive architectural survey may be found in Kusaba 1983). The church is cruciform in plan and vaulted throughout, with an internal length of 38.1 m and 35 m across the transepts. Detailed examination revealed four major phases of construction from *c.* 1160 to 1340: two twelfth-century campaigns including the building of the sacristy, choir,

crossing, transept arms, main arcade and part of the aisles. The two
western bays of the nave and remainder of the aisles and north porch date
to the first half of the thirteenth century. By 1340, with the completion of
the clerestory and high vault, the church of St Cross was more or less as it
stands now (**7**). John de Campedene, master 1382-1410, did much fine
work in the church, rebuilding the tower, reroofing the chancel and aisle,
installing a considerable amount of glazing and paving, enclosing the Lady
Chapel for the brethren and installing a high altar of alabaster and a
painted reredos. Thus a handsome building of considerable size, built to a
grand design with lavish architectural details, served as a magnificent
monument to ensure passage of the soul of Henry of Blois through
purgatory.

The project at St Cross was most ambitious and costly, yet Henry of
Blois and, more especially, his successors ensured that the standard of
work remained high throughout its lengthy period of construction. The
chapel at St Cross would always have been the focus of attention, the
finest building on the site. This emphasis on the chapel is also evident
at the more modest foundations. At Archbishop Lanfranc's hospital at
Harbledown (*c.* 1084) the chapel was distinguished by being the only
stone building on the site. It was described by Eadmer as 'a fair and large
house of stone' (Clay 1909: 196). In like manner the chapel of the hospital
of St Saviour, Bury St Edmunds, founded *c.* 1184, would have stood out
from its attached hall. An apartment at the eastern end of the hall, datable
to the latter part of the twelfth century, contained work of a quality
superior to the rest: the internal angles were of dressed stone and the
external angles finished with narrow buttresses of the same material. This
apartment may be identified with the chapel of St Thomas mentioned in
the accounts of 1386-7 (Burden 1925-9).

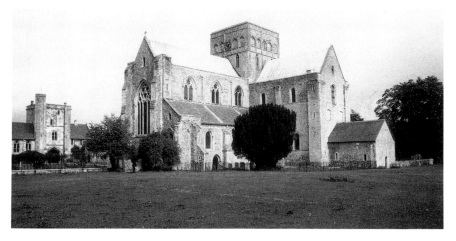

7 Church of the hospital of St Cross, Winchester; an impressive structure, begun in
the mid-twelfth century and completed by 1340.

As well as the hospital of St Saviour at Bury St Edmunds there also exists the partial remains of two other hospitals: St Petronilla, founded some time in the twelfth century, and St Nicholas, founded shortly before 1215. In both cases, of the whole it is only part of the chapel that remains. Their survival may, in part, be due to their continued use in some form or other at least until the Dissolution but it is more likely attributable to the high quality of their original construction.[1] Further, it is significant that at many other sites the only remains of the hospital are of its chapel, and so the more substantial nature of construction in comparison with the infirmary hall in underlined.

A fine example of a surviving twelfth-century chapel is the hospital of St Mary Magdalen, Stourbridge, Cambridgeshire, first recorded in 1169-72 for a master and lepers. The hospital ceased to function for lepers around 1279 but continued in use for worship up to the late fourteenth century. Despite a somewhat chequered career (it was used it turn as a storage place for the famous Stourbridge animal fair, a victualling house, a drinking booth, a stable and finally a barn), the chapel survived intact to illustrate the fine nature of work and high standards found in the chapels of even the smallest of foundations, forming one of the more 'complete and unspoilt pieces of Norman architecture' in the country (*VCH Cambridgeshire*: 133). The chapel of St Mary Magdalen was built on a small scale but occasionally even these humbler foundations had chapels which were constructed to quite ambitious designs. All that survives of the small leper hospital of St Giles, Maldon (8), founded *c*. 1164, for a warden, one chaplain and

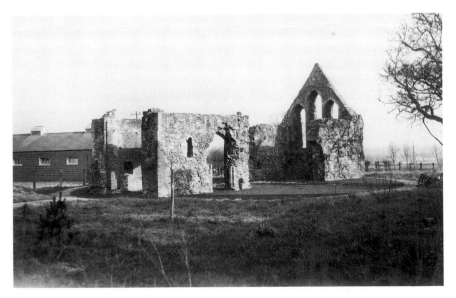

8   The chapel of the leper hospital, of St Giles, Maldon, built on a grand scale for such a small foundation.

leprous brethren, is part of the 'transepts' of a late-twelfth-century chapel obviously built on quite a grand scale to a size more than adequate for the nature of the foundation.

An example of a chapel from a later date at St Edmund's Hospital, Gateshead, founded *c*. 1247, shows these high standards continuing throughout the thirteenth century. The hospital was granted to the nuns of St Bartholomew's, Newcastle upon Tyne, in 1438 and was dissolved with the nunnery in 1539. It fortunately remained in a fair state of preservation until the south wall and west front of the chapel were incorporated into the new church of the Holy Trinity in 1837. The old chapel provides the newer church with a particularly fine west front with deeply recessed central doorway flanked by two tiers of arcades, while above these an upper arcade is pierced by lancets.

The chapels, in contrast to the infirmary halls, were subject to frequent attention, often resulting in quite major building alterations. Even the small chapel of the leper hospital at Harbledown, founded *c*. 1084, underwent a succession of modifications. Lanfranc's original church was a simple single-celled apsidal building which was replaced by a square-ended chancel soon after the archbishop's death. In the first half of the twelfth century a short north aisle was added and in the later twelfth or early thirteenth century a tower was built on to the end of the north aisle abutting the nave. In the fourteenth century the north aisle was extended to the east and a transeptal chapel added on the south. About the same time the Norman windows of the chancel were replaced and glazed.

Total rebuilding of the chapel, as at the hospital of St John the Baptist, Lichfield, in the mid-thirteenth century or at St John the Baptist, Northampton, in the early fourteenth century, was not uncommon. Elsewhere chapels were extended and enlarged, usually by the addition of a further chapel, as at the hospital of St Mary at Bath between 1310 and 1315 or at St Lazarus, St Martha and St Mary Magdalen, Sherburn, where a north chapel was added in 1316.

The chapel — the interior

The lasting quality of hospital chapel architecture as illustrated in the above examples is equalled by the character of the work found in the interiors of these chapels. A striking example is the chapel of God's House, Portsmouth, founded *c*. 1212. Although considerably restored, the interior provides an excellent example of the Early English style (9).

There are few remaining examples of the original schemes of hospital decoration. It is known that the hospital of St Mary at Ospringe possessed a clock in 1321-2, a rarity at this date in an establishment of such size. At Ospringe, and no doubt elsewhere, there would have been statues. But the only evidence comes from the chapel of the hospital of St John the Baptist, Coventry, where, on either side of the fine east window there survive the

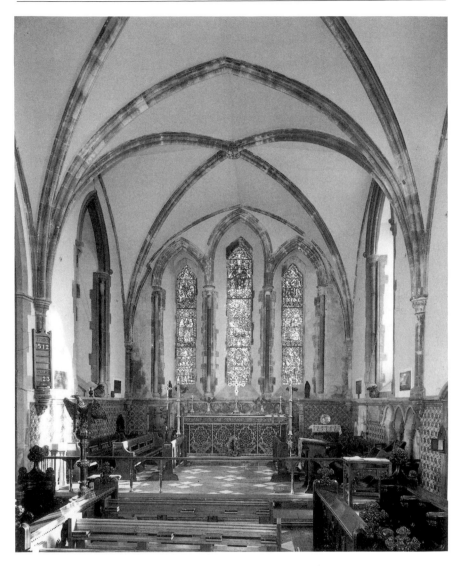

9 Fine quality work in Early English style at God's House, Portsmouth.

brackets upon which statues would have stood. A large wall-painting, datable to *c.* 1350, survives in the chapel of St Nicholas, Harbledown, depicting Mary and the Angel of Annunciation; also extant is a fine fourteenth-century stained-glass window with two figures of tiny censing angles bordered with fleurs-de-lis. There are traces of wall-paintings in the chapel of the small leper hospital of St Margaret and St Anthony at Wimborne, founded in the early thirteenth century, which suggest that this form of adornment may have been common even in the smaller foundations.

An intriguing glimpse of the chapel interior comes from the Newarke Hospital, Leicester. Here, two clerks were appointed to serve in the church and provide lights, vestments and vessels necessary for divine service. It would have been these clerks who changed the straw on the floor in winter or the rushes in summer, 'furnished out of the common fund ... as often as the church or its chancel be in need of such things' (Thompson 1937: 67). Elsewhere, inventories suggest that these chapels were well endowed in terms of vestments and plate.

The beginnings of change

More importantly, the Newarke Hospital illustrates the beginnings of the transition between the old-style infirmary-hall hospital and the foundations which were built or altered from the second half of the fourteenth century. Founded originally by Henry of Lancaster, *c.* 1350, and dedicated to the Annunciation of the Virgin Mary, the Newarke Hospital was greatly enlarged in 1351 by Henry's son, who joined to it a collegiate church, the whole then becoming known as the Newarke. Of the hospital buildings, the infirmary hall must have been most striking. Part of its fourteenth-century chapel remains and the nave and aisle can still be traced. The whole formed what must have been a magnificent hall, the largest of its kind, of seventeen bays, 67.1 m in length and still very much the standard design of infirmary hall with attached chapel. Housed in this hall, or 'nave', in the beds provided were thirty inmates of a temporary nature who were to be 'poor folk suffering from passing ailments who were to be examined by the warden before being granted relief' (Thompson 1937: 18).

But where the Leicester hospital differed from the earlier examples was in the special separate accommodation provided for the twenty *permanent* inmates, of the original constitution, chosen from those who could plead poverty, blindness or lameness, were stricken with palsy, had lost a limb, or were suffering from an incurable disease. Their accommodation was in a house adjoining the church, of which unfortunately no trace remains. Other buildings were also provided for the chaplains who were to reside for the duration of their lives and lead a common life in the hospital in the traditional manner and, more particularly, for the five nurses 'of good fame' (Thompson 1957: 17). These women were given a separate dwelling house also adjoining the church. There they remained until incapable of work; then the warden was to make provision for their living until one could succeed to a place in the almshouse. It was the requirement to make such a provision for retiring brethren that may have driven many foundations to take on the character of an almshouse (see Chapter III). But, as yet, at the Newarke attention was still focused on the infirmary hall, although separate dwellings were provided for each different class of resident, a change to be more greatly emphasized at a later date.

CHAPTER THREE

THE INFIRMARY-HALL TYPE
c. 1350-1547

By the beginning of the fourteenth century not only was the great age of
the building of the infirmary-hall type of hospital more or less over, but
many of the existing institutions were falling into decline. Pilgrimage was
beginning to lose its appeal and travellers were increasingly able to lodge
at inns. Furthermore the religious fervour which had inspired the foundation
of so many of the larger hospitals as well as the great monastic houses was
on the wane. Bequests fell away when the donor's allegiance changed in
favour of the smaller institutions of the parish church, friary and, significantly, the almshouse. The hospitals were no more immune to the other
economic problems of the early fourteenth century than their monastic
brethren, and they shared with them the growth in abuses in administration
and breakdown of monastic or religious life-style.

Nevertheless, some institutions survived and even prospered, carrying
out major alterations to their constitutions and, frequently, their buildings
to meet the changing conditions. This can be seen in contemporary
domestic architecture as well as the religious houses in the increased
provision of privacy and greater comfort. Hospitals which survived in this
period yet failed to meet these changing conditions continued with their
traditional way of life, maintaining the architectural emphasis on the
chapel, but they were doomed to failure at the Reformation.

The decline of the infirmary-hall type

Many hospitals be now for the most part decayed and the goods and
Profits of the same by divers Persons, as well Spiritual as Temporal,
withdrawn and spent in other Use ... Men and women have died
for lack of aid, livelihood and succour to the displeasure of God and
the peril of the souls of those who squander and misappropriate
the goods provided for these unfortunates by others (*Statutes of the
Realm* II: 175).

This was considered to be the state of the hospitals in 1414 and not
without reason. Facing both spiritual and economic decline, many hospitals
failed altogether or fell into ruin while others survived but were in a
parlous condition. A considerable number of foundations had degenerated

into free or chantry chapels. For example, the hospital of St John the Baptist, Buckingham, founded in the late thirteenth century, had by the end of the century become a chantry of St Thomas of Acon, London. There was little enthusiasm for the upkeep and maintenance of a property so distant, and when anticipated revenues failed to materialize, the foundation was allowed to fall into ruin. Other small foundations, like the hospital of St Mary Magdalen, Bawtry, founded some time before 1200, were never in effect more than chantries from the first. It was the fate of others, such as the hospital of St Nicholas and St Katherine of Canterbury, to fall into private hands, having survived a mere twenty-seven years.

Small foundations like St Nicholas and St Katherine of Canterbury were particularly at risk, as were many of the lazar houses, which were often small and poorly endowed. Decay and impoverishment in lazar houses at this time resulted from slender resources, diminishing revenues and maladministration rather than the disappearance of leprosy, although it had begun to decline in the mid fourteenth century. Many of these factors combined and caused the complete disappearance of numerous foundations; for example, the hospital of St Mary Magdalen, Winchester, left its mark in the architectural records only by the survival of its well, and at Tavistock the hospital is commemorated by a street name alone. Even the larger lazar houses found it difficult to maintain their original function. The leper hospital of Harbledown, founded at the end of the eleventh century for sixty inmates, supported only a few affected by the disease at the end of the fourteenth century (*Archaeological Journal* 86 (19: 29–30)). Similarly at the hospital of St Lazarus, St Martha and St Mary Magdalen at Sherburn, the largest leper hospital in the country built *c.* 1181 for the reception of sixty-five lepers, the statute of 1434 made provision for thirteen poor men and two lepers 'only if they could be found' (*VCH Durham* 2: 115).

Elsewhere some instances of destruction and dilapidation were due to outside causes. A raid by the French in 1338 burned down a considerable portion of God's House Hospital, Southampton. And by 1347, no doubt still suffering from the effects of the raid, the foundation needed to be

> quit of taxations, tallages, wools, custody and sea shore scutage, aids, grants, contributions and other charges to the king or his heirs by reason of lands and goods of the hospital (*CCh.R 1341–1417*: 30).

The hospital of St Mary Magdalen at Ripon also suffered badly from a raid, this time by the Scots. Not only was the foundation granted relief from taxation between 1315 and 1319 on account of its destruction, but in 1317 it was forced to turn away lepers. The Scots also raided the hospital of St Giles, Kepier, Durham in 1306, destroying the muniment room, damaging other property and crops, and leaving the foundation in a depressed state.

Nevertheless St Giles Hospital, perhaps fearing another raid but certainly heedless of the financial plight of the foundation, spent considerable funds on the building of a splendid two-storeyed gatehouse *c.* 1314 (**10**). But by 1355, the hospital was in such straits that an indulgence had to be granted to anyone who would contribute to the relief of the hospital, and by the mid fifteenth century revenues had fallen so seriously that they were not sufficient for the 'maintenance, building and repair of its houses' (Meade 1968: 51).

Over-ambitious building programmes, like that at St Giles, put severe strains on the resources of the early infirmary-hall type of foundation at this time and caused even the larger, better endowed institutions to run into serious debt. This is well illustrated at the hospital of St Thomas the Martyr, Canterbury, where a programme of repairs to the infirmary hall and the extension of its chapel in the early fourteenth century stretched the hospital's resources to the limit. Grants of protection are recorded in 1334, 1336 and again in 1353 when it was stated that they had 'not enough to live on unless relieved by the charitable collection of alms' (*CPR 1330–34*: 527, 559; *1334–38*: 306; *1350–54*: 529). The hospital was forced to appeal to the pope in 1363 for the grant of an indulgence for those 'visiting the chapel of St Mary the Virgin in the poor hospital of Canterbury, commonly called 'Estbridge ...' (*CPL 1362–1404*: 473).

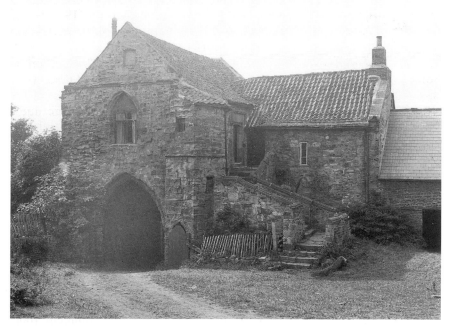

10 The ambitious gatehouse, added in the early fourteenth century to the hospital of St Giles, Kepier, Durham.

The major hospital of St Mary's, Dover, also found itself in great difficulty in the fourteenth century. Once again its problems coincided with a building project. An ambitious addition to its structure had been carried out in the early fourteenth century, a construction upon which little expense could have been spared. It is therefore not surprising to find the hospital in need of protection in the years 1313, 1317, 1325 and 1331 (*CPR 1307-13*: 583; *1313-17*: 622; *1327-30*: 160; *1330-34*: 71). By 1347, the brethren were in such dire circumstances that they complained to the king that 'they were reduced to such poverty that they cannot support themselves' and in 1375, the foundation was 'quit of all tallages, as they were bowed down in misfortune . . .'. This exemption from taxation was only the last of several granted during the fourteenth century (*CClR 1374-77*: 126, 551−2).[1]

Another large foundation which ran into difficulty in the fourteenth and early fifteenth centuries was St Leonard's Hospital, York. Extensive and costly work on some parts of the building clearly forced the neglect of other areas: known periods of construction are followed shortly afterwards by reports of dilapidation. In 1309, the dwelling house had been extended but by 1350 it was said to be in 'great disrepair' (*CPR 1348-50*: 518). Between 1364 and 1376 the foundation was ordered to provide a building divided into thirteen *studia* where the brethren might study the Holy Scriptures, and they were also to prepare a building for nursing mothers and infants. But by 1376-7 the commissioners were recording defects in the church, tower and dormitory. In 1400 an indulgence was granted for 'all who give alms for the repair and conservation of the fabric of the chapel of St Katherine . . .' (*CPL 1396-1404*: 340), at about the same time as a stone tower was added to the south end of the hospital. Yet in 1402 another report revealed many defects in the lead roof of the church and essential repairs were lacking to the roof of the infirmary house of the poor folk. At St Leonard's, the financial difficulties evidently persisted, for the buildings were again reported to be in ruin in the late fifteenth century.

A similar situation existed at St Mary's Hospital, Chichester, where in 1382, less than 100 years after the building of its fine infirmary hall, a commission was set up to inquire into the defects of the house, including buildings and furnishings. It is not recorded whether the buildings were indeed repaired but they were certainly described as in ruin again by the late fifteenth century (Wright 1885). Building campaigns begun in a spirit of optimism and exultation ended in impoverishment and, as the examples at York and Chichester show, once a foundation found itself in trouble it was extremely difficult, during the fourteenth century, to make a recovery, leading to a downward spiral of neglect and dilapidation.

One of the reasons for failure to recover was the general falling off in benefactions, particularly noticeable from the end of the thirteenth century. The majority of the infirmary-hall type of foundation had acquired most of their estates by this date, as had St Bartholomew's Hospital, Gloucester, where benefactions had more or less ceased by the mid-fourteenth century when the foundation was already reported as 'much decayed' (Ellis 1929: 192). Furthermore, when support for a hospital did continue, benefactions were likely to be small. One such example is the Commandery Hospital at Worcester where a number of small benefactions failed to save the foundation from pleading poverty in 1368 (*VCH Worcestershire* 2: 175). Even the previously much favoured St Mary's, Dover, found itself lacking support from its royal patron. Apart from grants of protection and exemption from taxation the few grants received in the later thirteenth and fourteenth centuries were less than generous in comparison with the privileges and favours granted to them in the earlier thirteenth century. Royal support for other foundations was also growing rarer in the fourteenth century.

St Mary's Hospital, Dover, also suffered from a long succession of corrodians (recipients of some form of maintenance) imposed upon it by the king. The practice whereby corrodians received board and lodging for life was common in the Middle Ages, and there are many examples of corrodians being imposed upon a foundation by its patron as a means of providing a pension or reward for old retainers. This type of provision for old retainers or relatives brought no financial gain and must have cost many an institution dearly. The hospital of St Mary Magdalen and St John the Baptist, Ely, can have been less than happy to receive the widow of one of the dependants of the Bishop of Ely in 1295. For a fee of a mere five marks the bishop bought free board and lodgings for the widow to include an ample daily diet of 9 litres of the better sort of ale, two loaves of bread and twice as much cooked meat as any brother had (Cobbett and Palmer 1936: 85). In 1316 the Bishop of London had 'condemned the great diminution of hospital funds through the reckless granting out of corrodies' at St Bartholomew's Hospital (Rawcliffe 1984: 4). The bishop forbade the further granting of corrodies without his consent but such exhortations rarely had any effect.

Corrodies depleted resources already scarce but a more serious result of the sale of corrodies was the growing tendency to discriminate among applications, with more beds reserved for longer-term occupants or paying guests than for the traditional wayfarers or pilgrims. Food, drink and accommodation were diverted from those in most need. Archbishop Stratford attempted to halt this trend at the hospital of St Thomas the Martyr, Canterbury, in 1342, when he decreed that

> poor pilgrims in good health shall be entertained for one night only ... that greater regard be had for the sick than the well pilgrims ... (Clay 1909: 167).

But at St Leonard's, York, in 1399, 97 out of 223 inmates had paid an entry fee, the master having sold corrodies in large numbers as well as the liveries of the sick and given them to esquires, merchants and well-to-do clerks. These practices inevitably led to the replacement of the sick and genuine bedesmen by the able-bodied, and consequent loss by the foundation of its eleemosynary purpose.

A greater evil than the sale of corrodies and of greater consequence for the fabric of a hospital, was the alienation of property and waste of goods. Hospitals and religious houses all over Europe faced problems with the poor administration of revenues. The papal bull *Quia Contingit*, issued by Pope Clement V (1305-16) for the hospitals and aimed at remedying the misappropriation, waste and negligence that were becoming widespread, seems to have had little effect. There are many examples of commissions set up to investigate maladministration. Such commissions were carried out at St Bartholomew's Hospital, Gloucester, in 1344, 1355, 1356 and 1358 but obviously to no avail, for by 1380 the foundation was in a scandalous state, the prior and brethren having taken away the beds of the poor and after death appropriating their clothing. They had also made a great door in the house of the poor through which they carried hay and drove pigs. Further commissions were set up at Gloucester in 1381, 1382, and 1384 (Ellis 1929: 201-2).

The hospital of St John the Baptist, Northampton, was also brought close to ruin by the behaviour of the brethren. In 1382, Bishop Buckingham complained that at a recent visitation the brethren

> foolhardily spend, waste and publicly dilapidate the goods and rents and profits of the aforesaid house, so that, while within a short space they unadvisedly consume their future means of life, they must be drawing near utter want and destruction and ruin ... (Seymour 1947: 157).

The hospital survived, although not without considerable changes to its constitution and buildings.

Another hospital faced by similar difficulties, but which did lose its independence and finally its existence, was St Mary's at Ospringe. In 1330 the king had commissioned a visitation which reported the house 'to be greatly decayed by lack of good rule' (Drake 1914: 51). The prosperity of the house was clearly in decline again in the fifteenth century when, in 1413, a visitation inquired into waste by the improvident governance of wardens or masters and was followed by further inquiries into bad governance in 1418, 1422 and 1458 (Drake 1914: 56-60).

Apart from Ospringe, there are numerous other instances of irregularities or dishonesty of wardens and masters. This inevitably led to a reduction in the quality and quantity of the food distributed to the staff and the infirm. At St Katherine's Hospital, Ledbury, in 1398, it was found that owing to the negligence of the master, the brothers and sisters had been so badly supplied with food that they had been driven '*ad mendicandum panem, ad scandalum hospitalis predicti*' (to begging for bread, bringing scandal to the hospital) (Bannister 1918-20: 65). The master at Ledbury was non-resident and had probably appropriated the revenues of the hospital for his own use.

The absorption of the greater part of a hospital's revenues by the brethren and sisters and, more particularly, the master or warden, increased throughout the fourteenth and fifteenth centuries. God's House, Southampton, serves as a typical example. Up to the fourteenth century, much of the charitable expenditure had been directed towards the resident poor, but from 1328, less was expended upon the infirm than the staff – there was a reduction in the quantity of bread baked and a marked change in the quality, although fine white bread was purchased for the warden's visits. At this time, the warden, Gilbert de Wyggeton, the king's nominee, was an absentee. But on all his visits the warden received better meals than did even the brethren and sisters; the accounts show that wine was hardly ever purchased except when the warden was in residence, fresh meat was also brought in with far greater frequency on these occasions, as was the purchase of a wider variety of fresh fish, fruit and species. When de Wyggeton did reside at the hospital for any length of time he was a great burden on the hospital's finances; the hospital accounts reveal some of the comfort which masters and their relatives received from these institutions. In 1328-9, Gilbert de Wyggeton resided at the hospital for forty-three days. On his departure his relative, William de Wyggeton, remained. This William had expensive tastes in chicken, fresh fish and pomegranates (Harris 1970).

Not only did wardens and masters reduce the consumable resources of a hospital but many also regarded the movables as for their personal disposal. No better example can be found than St Bartholomew's Hospital, Gloucester where, in 1380, at great detriment to the buildings, the prior and brethren had unroofed a great house (hall) of the poor and taken the timber and tiles for their own use. The pillage apparently continued, for in 1359 it was reported that money, corn, jewels, silver and brass vessels, bed and household utensils worth £100, which had been given to the hospital by the men of Gloucester and elsewhere, were alleged to have been dissipated and destroyed (*CPR 1358-61*: 224). Furnishings and vestments of the well-stocked chapel provided even greater pickings. In 1418 the commissioners at Ospringe were ordered to inquire into the dispersion, sale and abduction of many relics, ornaments, books and jewels by the master and executors (*CPR 1416-22*: 208).

Similar examples of bad management and negligence occurring elsewhere put the domestic buildings particularly at risk. One of the worst instances of dilapidation of buildings due to abuse by the masters was that of St Cross Hospital, Winchester. An almost unbroken succession of corrupt masters governed St Cross Hospital from the early fourteenth century. A series of disastrous appointments to the mastership due either to nepotism or favouritism resulted in the funds being diverted from their original purpose and the number of inmates being much reduced, causing almost total ruin. From time to time the Bishop of Winchester took the situation in hand as did Bishop Asserio in carrying out commissions of inquiry into the defects of the house in 1321. There was apparently little success, for in 1332 a report described the goods of the house as 'dilapidated' (Cave 1970: 10). By 1336 the buildings had collapsed and were in a ruinous condition. Improvements were carried out at this date and other buildings were repaired in 1375–6. In 1372, the government of the hospital was finally taken over by William of Wykeham (Bishop of Winchester 1367-1404). The condition of the hospital by the end of the fourteenth century is revealed in an account of the proceedings taken by Bishop Wykeham against the master, Roger Clun, who had sold the cattle, the corn, materials, had turned out the brethren, refused to render accounts and embezzled the profits of the house and allowed the buildings to fall into decay. Wykeham recorded that the great hall had fallen in and 100 poor men fed there daily had been removed to a 'hovel' at the gate. Other buildings had been pulled down by a previous master and the thirteen permanent inmates ejected. Furthermore, the church, begun in the early twelfth century, was still unfinished (Cave 1970: 13).

The domestic buildings of St Cross Hospital were saved by William of Wykeham's nominee to the mastership, John de Campedene. Although a personal friend of the bishop, de Campedene, upon taking up office, was made to swear an oath

> to make a faithful inventory of the goods of the same House, and duly administer the same goods, and also annually to render a reasonable and true account thereof, according to the requirements aforesaid (Cave 1970: 13).

Although little trace remains of the domestic buildings of this date, true to his word de Campedene kept a careful record of his expenditure. Apart from the details expended on books, vestments and plate, the amount handed to the steward each year 'for the necessary repairs and expenses of this house' is listed. By 1407, before the costly vaulting of the nave, this amounted to £1,980 5s. 6d., much of which must have come from his own purse *'de bonis suis propriis'* (Carr 1960).

The chapels c.1350–c.1547

St Cross Hospital, Winchester, was fortunate, indeed, in its master. The crowning glory of de Campedene's achievement must be accounted its chapel. Following the tradition of the early infirmary-hall type of foundation, the emphasis at St Cross remained with the ecclesiastical buildings. De Campedene's main work was on improvement and completion of the chapel where he rebuilt the tower and increased its height, and roofed the chancel and aisles. He also constructed the lantern and installed a considerable amount of glazing in the lantern and triforia of the choir. He entirely remodelled the interior of the church, putting in stalls and paving as well as setting up, in 1385, a splendid altarpiece of alabaster. His greatest achievement was the revaulting of the nave in *c.* 1407-10 ensuring, at last, the completion of the church begun by Henry de Blois (**11**). As a tribute to his achievement, a monumental brass of John de Campedene now lies under the tower, consisting of a full-length figure of the master in his ecclesiastical robes with hands raised in prayer (**12**).

Since the chapel remained the focus of attention it is there that most evidence of building activity occurs after *c.* 1350. At Norwich, Bishop Spencer completely rebuilt the chapel of St Giles Hospital in 1380 despite its already considerable size. The pre-eminence of the chapel was emphasized by the provision of a magnificent interior. The outstanding feature is its wagon roof, built of chestnut and adorned with 252 double-headed eagles in the panel representing the emblem of the Holy Roman Empire, said to have been so decorated as a compliment to Queen Anne of Bohemia, daughter of Charles of Prague and wife of Richard II, who is reputed to have visited Norwich at the time of the reconstruction of the chapel. The chapel was also provided with a great new east window which retains its very fine tracery and some of the original stained glass (**13**). Other good windows survive on the north; those of the south are now lost.

St Giles Hospital was exceptional. Construction work, even to the chapels, had more or less come to a halt by the end of the fifteenth century. Nevertheless, surviving documentary evidence shows that the chapels were still well maintained. The accounts of 1512 for the Holy Trinity Hospital, Bristol, founded in 1395, reveal a clean, cared-for chapel, with frequent entries for lamp oil, tapers, new wax, scouring the standards, scouring the lamps before the altar, and for rushes (Pritchard 1911: 93).

Inventories such as these show chapels to have been continually well equipped. By 1535, St Mary's Hospital, Dover, was still well provided for with the vestry containing candlesticks, cruets, censers, an incense-boat, corporas, copes, vestments, three carpets of tapestry to be laid before the altar, two carpets of red wool and two of white wool and three other carpets to be laid before altars, two cushions made of an old cope and two other cushions (Walcott 1868: 296-7). Even as late as the reign of Edward VI, St John's Hospital, Canterbury, could still boast robes of black and red velvet, white fustian and a cope of Bruges satin (Clay 1909: 165). Very likely St John's would once have been as well equipped as was St Cross Hospital, Winchester, in 1383 when twenty-one chasubles, twenty-seven albs, twenty-five stoles, besides other necessary items were listed in an inventory. Such items were frequently the gifts of benefactors to the foundation. At St Cross, it was the master John de Campedene who not only restored the buildings but also contributed greatly to the stock of

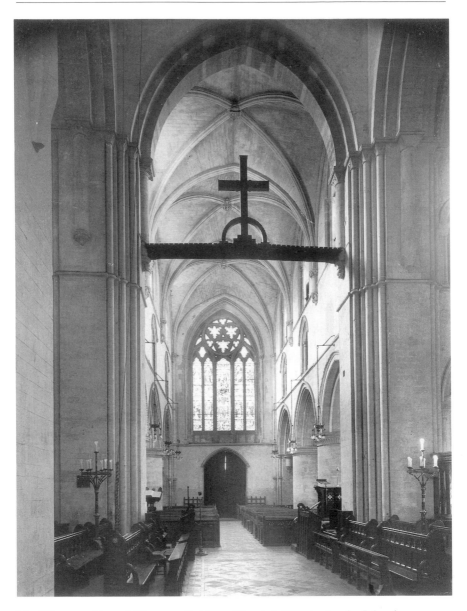

11 The revaulting of The nave St Cross Hospital, Winchester, by John de Campedene in 1340 completed the church begun by Henry de Blois in the mid-twelfth century.

vestments, books and plate, recording in detail the cost and materials used for each item (Carr 1960: 21).

Thus the chapels did not suffer such neglect in their later years as did the domestic buildings. But complete rebuildings, quite common in the

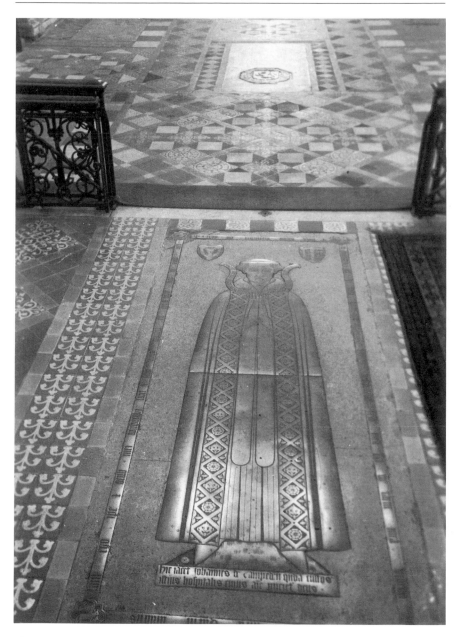

12   Monumental brass of John de Campedene, in the church of St Cross, master and great benefactor to the hospital at Winchester.

earliest period, were, from the late fourteenth century, quite rare. Exceptions included the chapel of Abbot Bere's almshouse at Glastonbury, founded *c.* 1512, a relatively plain and modest structure **(14)**, and the more

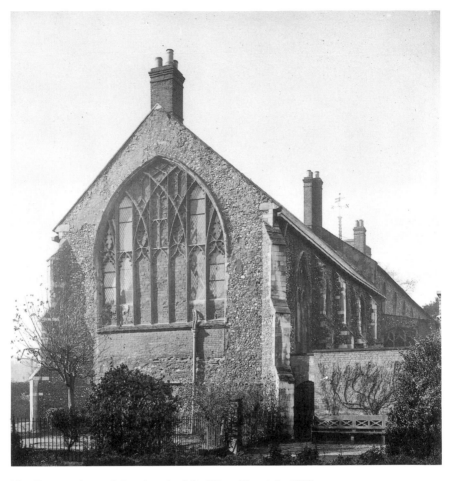

13   East window, of the chapel of St Giles, Norwich, 1380.

splendid edifice, in keeping with the tradition of fine chapel building, to be found at St Mark's Hospital, Bristol **(15, 16)**.

St Mark's Hospital, founded *c.* 1220, followed the typical pattern of development of the early hospital foundations described in Chapter I. The nave dates from *c.* 1230 and was enlarged in the 1260s by the addition of the south aisle and chapel. Again, in common with other large foundations, there is no evidence of construction work during the fourteenth and early fifteenth centuries. At the end of the fifteenth century a tower was constructed and in the early sixteenth century much work took place in the chancel chapel due to the benefaction of Miles Salley, Bishop of Llandaff. Bishop Salley equipped the chapel with a fine altarpiece (now much restored) and four elaborately carved sedilia. Bishop Salley died in 1516

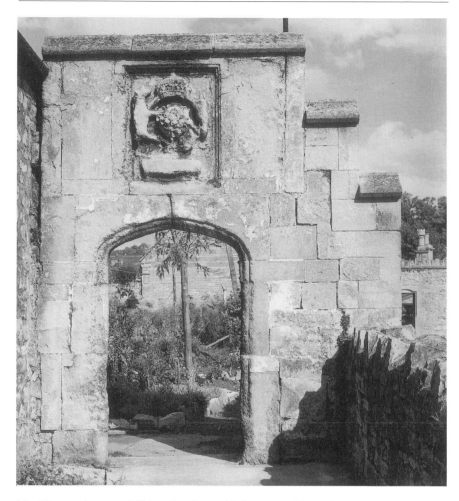

14 The gatehouse, of Abbot Bere's establishment at Glastonbury. a more modest foundation of the early sixteenth century.

and was buried in the chapel; his tomb occupied the north-east corner of the chancel, a position most often favoured by founders and great benefactors.[2] Adjoining the bishop, and also attributed to his munificence, is the equally magnificent canopied monument of Sir Thomas Berkeley (died 1316) and his lady (**17**).

The fine chapel of Bishop Salley was far surpassed in splendour with the addition of another chapel by the benefaction of Sir Robert Poyntz of Iron Acton. Sir Robert was connected by marriage to the Berkeleys and through them to the Gaunts (founders and benefactors of the hospital). He was also a prominent member of the courts of Henry VII and Henry VIII. Shortly before his death in 1520 he ordained that he should be buried in

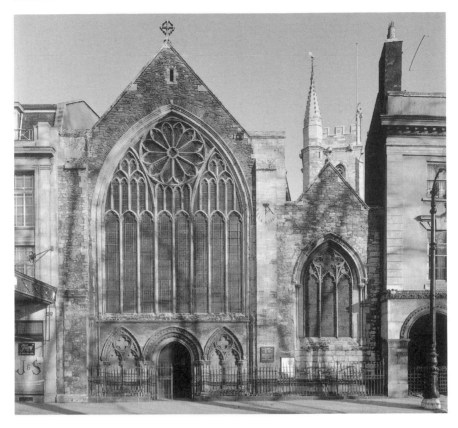

15 St Mark's, Bristol. Continual reconstruction from the late twelfth century maintained the fine tradition of chapel building.

> the church of the Gaunts' beside Bristol in the chapel of Jesus which latter I have caused to be newly edified and made at my cost and charges, on the south side of the chancel of the said church and the over part thereof behind the presbytery there ... (Cook 1947: 183).

Provision for Sir Robert's chapel, known as the Poyntz chapel, was extravagant as the instructions to his executors reveal:

> The said new chapel which I lately edified is not in all things perfect and finished yet according to mine intent, that is to wit, the glazing of the windows there are making of two pews within the said chapel in the lower end of the same, mine executors shall finish and perform all the things being yet undone and shall also garnish the same chapel and certain images and the altar of the same with altar cloths, vestments, books and chalices and all other things thereunto necessary ... (Cook 1947: 183).

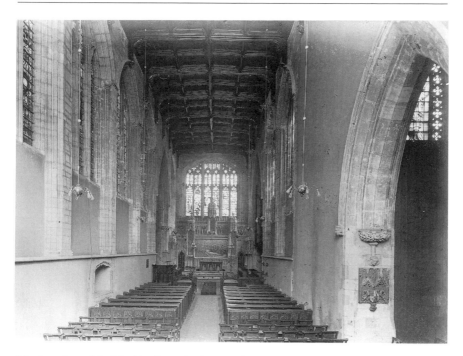

16 Interior of St Mark's, Bristol, showing fine workmanship.

Sir Robert's executors evidently completed his design in fine style by 1536 — the date on the east window at Iron Acton.

The Jesus or Poyntz chapel is an impressive late chantry chapel and is a fine example of the architecture of that date. The ornate detail and delicacy of the design and stonework suggest that Sir Robert employed the designer commissioned by Bishop Salley for his work in the chancel. Its most notably attractive and beautiful feature is the fan vault on which are carved the arms of Henry VIII and Catherine of Aragon along with those of the founder and his wife Margaret Woodville (**18**). Sir Robert's 'vestments, books and chalices' were an important part of the fitting out of the chapel and in comparison with the sparse nature of the contents of the infirmary hall, chapels were well provided for. Sir Robert had provided his chapel with a series of sixteenth-century wall-paintings, the floor was paved with enamelled tiles from Spain interspersed with a few English encaustic tiles bearing heraldic devices, and several elaborately canopied niches, once holding images, adorned the walls.

The masters' houses

Apart from the chapels, another group of buildings singled out for special attention, particularly from the fifteenth century, were the dwellings provided for the master or warden. Similar provision of private dwellings for abbots

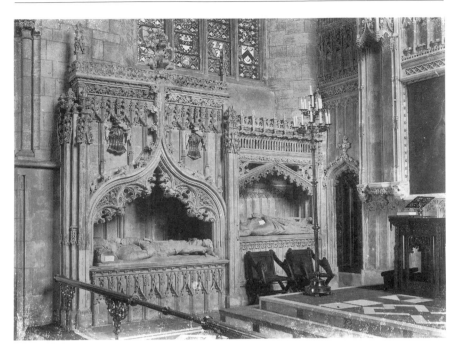

17 Monuments to Bishop Miles Salley and Sir Thomas Berkeley, benefactors to St Mark's Hospital, Bristol, situated in a favoured place in the chancel.

can also be found in the religious houses of this date. By the time of the Reformation a number of hospital foundations would have had a master's house which could have been described, like that of the hospital of St Bartholomew, Gloucester, as a 'fayre lodging' (as described by Leland, quoted in Ellis 1929: 190).

These entirely separate dwellings can be seen as originating in the desire by the masters for some form of privacy, datable from at least as early as the beginning of the fourteenth century. The original statutes of the earliest foundations obliged the master to sleep and eat in common with the brethren. By the beginning of the fourteenth century these statutes were clearly being violated; for example, in 1315 the master of St Giles Hospital, Durham, had to be reminded of his communal obligations and was only declared exempt from them if he was in attendance upon the bishop (Meade 1968: 51). By this date the master at Durham almost certainly occupied a private apartment as did the master of the hospital of St John the Baptist and St Mary Magdalen, Ely, by 1303 when he was forbidden to dine alone in his private room (Cobbett and Palmer 1936: 82).

Once a private room for the master was commonplace, the need for increased privacy and more special provision grew. It may have taken the form of a solar wing, as seen at St Mary's, Canterbury, or more substantial

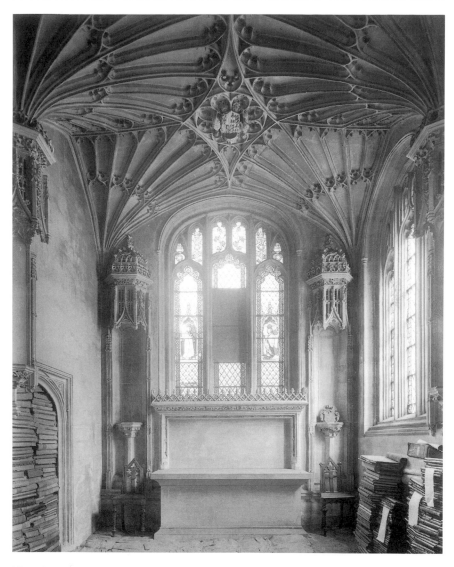

18   The Jesus or Poyntz chapel within St Mark's Hospital, Bristol, a rare example of fine chapel building in the sixteenth century.

alterations to the fabric, as at St Cross Hospital, Winchester, when, in 1336, the master is recorded as building, or at least altering, part of the premises (possibly the hall) to be used as chambers for the master (Woodward 1974: 230). This house was further improved and added to in 1393 for the comfort of the Earl of Kent who stayed there during the parliament held in Winchester that year. With the building of Cardinal Beaufort's Almshouse of Noble Poverty at St Cross, the master took up a new, even finer residence in the gatehouse.

As at St Cross Hospital, the master of the hospital of St John the Baptist at Northampton also chose to be entirely separate from the brethren by the appropriation and conversion of the refectory which stood a little to the north-east of the infirmary hall and chapel (1, 20). The earliest work in the building (now demolished) dated from the early thirteenth century. Considerable alterations were carried out in the late fifteenth and early sixteenth centuries, improving the building by the partitioning of rooms and insertion of chimneys. This increase of privacy and comfort probably marked the date of occupation by the master (Dryden 1873-4: 228).

The master of St Katherine's Hospital, Ledbury, also built himself a fine residence, separate from but alongside the infirmary hall. The master's house dates from the fifteenth century, when it consisted of one range with a kitchen and solars at east and west ends. What is especially interesting at Ledbury is the survival of the two buildings, which enables their dimensions to be compared. The master's house in the fifteenth century measured almost 18 m. In contrast, only 24 m were allocated to the inmates of the infirmary hall. The master's house was further improved and extended in the sixteenth and seventeenth centuries when the accounts show the house to be alive with continual building activity with the constant employment of carpenters, glaziers, plumbers, joiners, masons, pargeters, smiths, tilers and thatchers. The former solar wing was lined

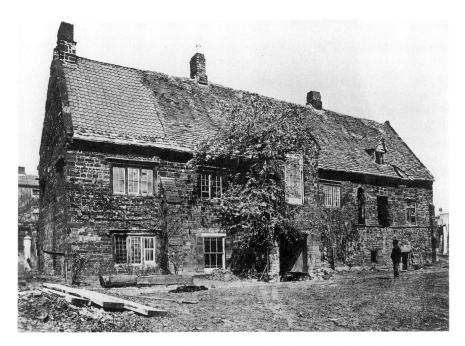

19   The master's house of St John the Baptist, Northampton before demolition.

with panelling and a frieze; the fireplace was flanked by Ionic pilasters and the overmantel was graced by a painting of Bishop Foliot (Bannister 1918-20: 65).

Changes to the infirmary-hall type

Changes in privacy and comfort for the masters were soon passed on to the brethren and sisters and also came to be expected for the inmates. The rule, as laid down for many of the infirmary-hall type of institution, stated that common dormitories and refectories were to be used. This arrangement was typified by the hospital of St John the Baptist, Abingdon, where the accounts of the abbey almoner revealed that the hospital consisted of a chamber for the brethren, a chamber for the sisters, a chapel and dormitory for the sick (*Med. Arch.* 1968: 56). Nevertheless, the ideas of increased privacy and comfort, much in contravention of the spirit of the rule, but as seen already in the separate apartments and houses of the wardens and masters, and also to be found in the infirmaries of the religious houses, soon extended to all other classes of inmate, and became a special feature of the hospitals and almshouses after *c.* 1350.

Separation of the sexes in one form or another was common enough, but another form of differentiation was also practised. Within these institutions it seems that some form of preferential treatment for certain classes (apart from the masters) had always existed. In particular, it was not uncommon for the priests or certain other distinguished brethren to be given special privileges. The priests of the hospitals of St Mary, Chichester, and St Bartholomew, Gloucester, were regarded as the most honoured brethren next to the master and as such were to be given 'fitting' residences within the hospital (Wright 1885: 20; Ellis 1929: 189). At St Giles Hospital, Norwich, it was the poor chaplains of the diocese 'broken down with age or destitute of bodily strength, or labouring under continual disease' who were to be received into the hospital and given suitable board and lodgings in an 'honourable part of the house' (*VCH Norfolk*: 443). Other high-ranking hospital officials probably also had their own chambers, as did, for example, the cellarer at St Leonard's Hospital, York, as early as 1294 (*VCH Yorkshire* 3: 337).

Just what this preferential treatment was is difficult to determine. But St Leonard's, York, was the largest foundation of its kind, and at the larger hospitals there would almost certainly have been private chambers or even special buildings set aside for the patron and important guests. The excavations at St Mary, Ospringe, have provided a very good idea of what one such building was like. In a small close to the north-east of the infirmary hall, within the hospital precinct, stood a group of buildings comprising a substantial stone-built first-floor hall and adjoining it were two more small rooms and another building with an undercroft. This close of buildings was constructed shortly after the infirmary hall, and the fine quality of the remains, including painted wall-plaster, decorated tiles and window glass as well as first-floor fireplaces, suggest that this was probably the building constructed for the use of Henry III and later occupied by Edward I and Edward II upon their visits to Ospringe. This building came later to be known as the *camera regis*. A similar set of buildings probably existed at St Mary's, Dover, another foundation of Henry III, where the chancellor was entitled to livery for himself and for the clerks of the chancery.

Where there was no special provision, fine chambers might have been set aside for the royal and other important secular guests who visited the hospitals, such as those received at St Giles, Kepier, Durham, where accommodation was provided for both Edward I and Queen Isabella and similarly at God's House, Southampton, upon receiving Margaret of Anjou and her retinue for four days on their arrival in England. Other foundations also provided, as did the religious houses, for gentlefolk boarders. Lady Jane Guildford described her abode at St Mark's Hospital, Bristol, in 1535 as 'a lodging, chosen as meet for a poor widow to serve God' (*VCH Gloucestershire* 2: 117) and accommodation of such a standard would no doubt have been found at St Bartholomew's Hospital, London, where rents were received for houses in the grounds; the house adjoining the Smithfield gate facing the chapel was occupied in the fifteenth century by Lady Joan Astley, nurse of Henry VI, while the Recorder of London and Clerk of Works also lived in the hospital at the same time.

Corrodians, like Lady Jane Guildford and Lady Joan Astley, were not always detrimental to the well-being of a foundation. Such corrodians were usually required to present gifts of land or funds to a community before entry. A decent chamber would have been prepared at St Bartholomew's Hospital, Gloucester, in 1220, for Sir Henry Berkeley who had released land to the hospital in return for being received into the community. Sir Henry died shortly afterwards, causing little expense, but considerable gain, to the foundation (Ellis 1929: 193). It is not known what James le Palmere of London gave to the hospital of St Mary, Dover, for entry into their community in 1360, but he was to occupy 'the new chamber in the hospital over the larder and upon the water flowing there opposite the prior of Dover's watermill for life' (*CPR 1358-61*: 512). Palmere or his patron may have provided the hospital with sufficient funds for the buildings of the chamber, and he was only one of a long list of successive corrodians received at the Dover hospital in the fourteenth century.

Corrodians like Sir Henry Berkeley and James le Palmere must have had certain expectations for their life-style within these foundations, and such occupants may have prompted the increase in private chambers particularly noticeable in the hospitals from the end of the fourteenth century. Indeed, by 1535 the Dover hospital possessed a considerable variety of private apartments, as detailed in an inventory of that date:

... the Great Chamber called the Hoostrye ... the Littlell Chamber
within the Hoostrye ... one other Littlell Chamber ... the chamber
Over the Water [probably that occupied by James le Palmere] ... the
Chamber within that ... another Littlell chamber within that ... the
Chamber called Sir Peers' Chamber ... the Master's chamber ...
(Walcott 1868: 277-9).

The identification of 'Sir Peers' is not known but he must have been a
gentleman of some consequence or a great benefactor. He almost certainly
would have demanded a high standard of comfort and considerable privileges, probably much akin to those received by Sir Philip Wem at Ospringe.
Sir Philip Wem was Rector of Crundale but by 1401 was occupying the
'chamber situated by the garden gate of the hospital on the west side'. He
was also provided with considerable comforts. Each week he was entitled
to have the food allowances of two senior brethren; he was to be provided
with a livery of woollen cloth yearly as good 'as the best brother has'; the
master and brethren were also to carry to his chamber two cartloads of
their wood for his fuel and he should have six pounds of candles for his
chamber. The master and brethren were also to repair the chamber and
keep it 'wynthyt' and watertight. Sir Philip and his servants were also
allowed free ingress and egress at the chamber, kitchen, brewhouse and
bakehouse (*CPR 1401-05*: 7).

Alongside the provision of private chambers for corrodians and rich
boarders, improvements were also made to the accommodation of the
ordinary brethren, sisters and inmates. This, too, took the form of an
increase in privacy. For example, excavations at St Mary's, Canterbury,
revealed a mass of post-holes representing extensive partitioning of the
hall which probably took place during the major building campaign of
c. 1370. Similar partitioning may also have taken place during the late-
fourteenth-century reconstruction of the hall and chapel of the small
hospital of St Mary, Strood. Neither hospital was a rich foundation, and
partitioning of the infirmary hall to provide greater privacy was possibly
one solution favoured by the smaller foundations, as certainly occurred in
contemporary religious houses.

One of these small foundations was the hospital of St Mary Magdalen
at Glastonbury. The thirteenth-century chapel was reroofed in the fourteenth century and possibly, at the same time, the infirmary hall was
partitioned. Further improvements to the infirmary hall took place in the
late fifteenth or sixteenth century when the hall roof was removed and the
cubicles converted into individual dwellings. The north and south rows
were separately roofed thus providing a narrow open courtyard down the
centre.

The hospital at Glastonbury may only have been able to afford the more
extensive renovations in making entirely separate apartments in its later
years. But many of the larger or richer foundations, upon rebuilding,

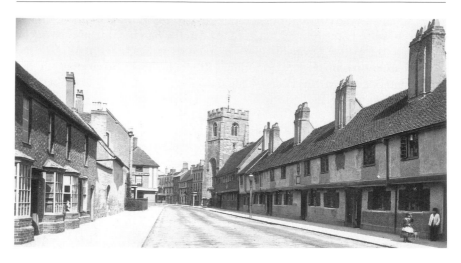

20   The almshouses of Holy Cross, Stratford-on-Avon, rebuilt as individual dwellings in *c.* 1427.

converted their infirmary halls directly into separate, individual apartments rather than go through the intermediate phase of partitioning. One of the earliest examples comes from the hospital of the Holy Cross at Stratford-upon-Avon (**20**). Here the hospital, founded in 1269, was rebuilt when it became part of Stratford College *c.* 1427. The structure, consisting of a range 45.7 m in length, was of ten bays of two storeys, the upper storey being jettied at the front, and provided individual accommodation for ten poor persons.

The rebuilding at Stratford coincided with a change in the organization of the foundation that virtually amounted to a refoundation. Very often it was such a refoundation that provided the impetus for a rebuilding programme, just as it did at the hospital of St John the Baptist, Lichfield, in 1495-6 (**21**). Bishop Smyth not only reformed the hospital and gave it fresh statutes but he also considerably improved the domestic buildings. The thirteenth-century chapel remained untouched but the adjoining infirmary hall was almost completely rebuilt and converted into a two-storeyed range with chimneys divided by a cross-passage to provide separate dwellings for thirteen poor men.

Another good example comes from the hospital of St John the Baptist, Northampton. The hospital was originally thought to have consisted of a large infirmary hall with aisles and connecting chapel (**22**). A rebuilding programme, probably in the early fourteenth century, although now only the west front is of that date, converted the south aisle into private chambers with a common hall. A similar reconstruction may have taken place at St Bartholomew's, Sandwich, founded *c.* 1190, where documentary evidence reveals that during the fourteenth century the brethren had

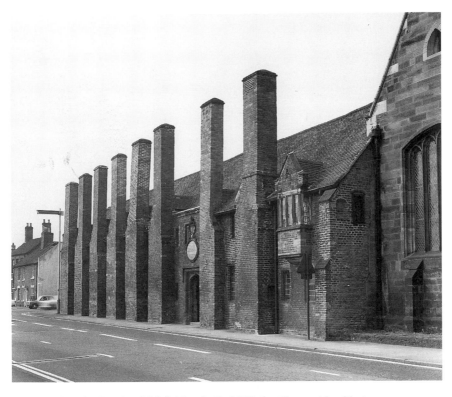

21 St John the Baptist, Lichfield, rebuilt 1495-6 with considerable improvements including the large chimneys still standing on the road side.

separate rooms although within one connected building retaining a communal hall, bakehouse and kitchen.

The structural changes which took place at St Bartholomew's, Sandwich, and also at St John the Baptist, Northampton, reflected changes in the nature of the foundation. At St Bartholomew's, by 1435, the brethren and sisters had become almsfolk, with the next vacancy being granted to a person in consideration of a sum of money. By this date the inmates at Sandwich were also more independent and self-sufficient, being granted money in lieu of food and drink yet still having a common pot into which each person was to put his or her own meat. No one was permitted use of a separate pot (Boys 1792: 6). At Northampton, hospital provision had to be made for the eight poor persons to be maintained as detailed by the bequest of John Dallington in 1340 (Dryden 1873-4: 228). This probably marks the date of the alterations and the time when the hospital became an almshouse, for it was certainly functioning as such in 1534 when eight persons were still being provided for (*Valor Ecclesiasticus* 4: 316).

A similar change in function may have prompted the major structural alterations which took place towards the end of the fifteenth century at the

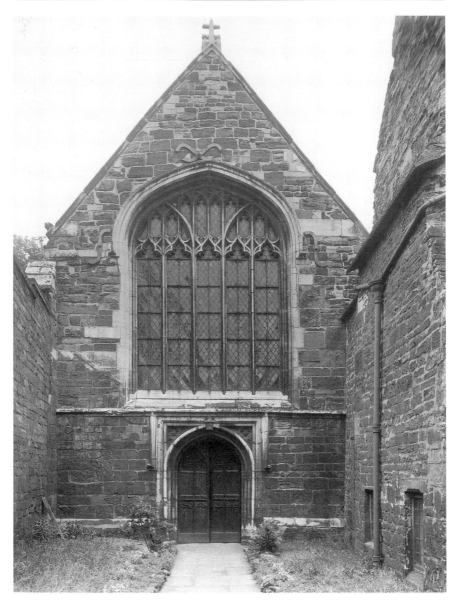

22 The chapel adjoining the infirmary hall of the hospital of St John the Baptist, Northampton, rebuilt along with much of the hospital in the early fourteenth century.

hospital of St Nicholas, Salisbury. By 1478, the brethren and sisters of St Nicholas were certainly classed as pensioners and the foundation had completely taken on the character of an almshouse. According to the foundation charter of 1245, the brethren had clear duties in the care of the sick and for the running of the establishment. Yet as early as 1250, several of the brethren were classed with the infirm (Wordsworth 1902: xlxi). Some form of special provision was obviously made for those brethren or sisters whose age or infirmity prevented them from carrying out their duties. What such provision was can be clearly seen at Salisbury in the fifteenth century when the original infirmary hall, with its central arcade and double chapel, was transformed. The south aisle was enclosed to make up the inmates' chambers and further individual rooms were built elsewhere on the site. The north porch was also turned into a separate tenement and the rooms above the south aisle were reserved for the use of the chaplains. The north chapel was converted into a common hall and the north aisle demolished in 1498. The starting date of this programme is probably marked by the granting of a request for a portable altar in March 1461-2 (*CPL 1455-64*: 627). The rededication of the chapel of St Nicholas in 1493 would probably signify the completion of the works. The south aisle had evidently been converted by 1478 when the statutes ordained that the brothers and sisters should not behave in their rooms or in hidden places in such a way as to arouse suspicion (Wordsworth 1902: lxii).

However, the relaxation of the rule by the provision of increased privacy, as seen at St Nicholas, Salisbury and elsewhere, may also have been responsible for concurrent and much criticized increases in the laxity of behaviour. The building of the individual chambers at the hospital of St John the Baptist, Northampton, was accompanied by reports of 'extravagances of food and clothing' of the brethren who were also enjoined to 'abstain from revelling and drinking parties' held in private chambers (injunctions of Bishop Buckingham, 1381, in Dryden 1873-4: 215-17). There were also frequent inquiries into infraction of the rule at St Katherine's, Ledbury, for example in 1535, when punishment was urged for '*Errores et excessus fratrum et conversorum* ...' (Bannister 1918-20: 65). The situation in 1364 at St Leonard's Hospital, York, had so deteriorated that a visitation ordered the setting aside of a special chamber in the house in which 'offending and incorrigible brothers could be maintained' (*VCH Yorkshire* 3: 339).

Thus the changing emphasis towards improvements in the domestic buildings by the provision of private chambers led to general relaxations of the rule, with ensuing difficulties, and must have added to the problems already presented to many of the hospitals by diminishing revenues and abuses in administration. Once the spiritual functions of the early foundations were eroded, many benefactors gave their support to the new types of foundation which sprang up in the later fourteenth and, more especially, the fifteenth centuries.

CHAPTER FOUR

THE LATE MEDIEVAL HOSPITAL: THE BEDEHOUSE

The decades of the mid fourteenth century marked a turning-point in hospital construction. Few new hospitals were founded in the years immediately following the Black Death. When building began again *c.* 1380 the new foundations, having adapted to changing conditions, served a definite purpose as long-term residences for almsfolk with all the increased privacy and comforts that such a resident would, by this date, have demanded. Indeed, there was rarely any provision for the sick. If an inmate of one of the new foundations was taken ill he was liable, as at Higham Ferrers, to be removed from the establishment until his recovery. It was not until the early sixteenth century that a new hospital, the Savoy in London, was founded especially to provide care for the temporary, sick inmate.

Within this new phase of foundation, two main types of bedehouse or almshouse arose. Some were built much in the tradition of the earliest hospitals. Plans of the surviving institutions at Higham Ferrers (1423), Wells (1424), Sherborne (1437) and Stamford (1475) bear a considerable resemblance, but on a smaller scale, to the earlier infirmary-hall type of design. Typically they consisted of a small narrow hall with terminating chapel under one roof. The hall was, from the first, divided into cubicles, a practice common by this date in contemporary monastic infirmaries and also seen to be taking place in the earlier hospital foundations.

Alongside the new infirmary-hall type of foundation, however, were built a completely different set of establishments. These foundations were characteristically, although not exclusively, quadrangular in plan, consisting of groups of lodgings, a chapel and refectory surrounding an open courtyard, as seen at Arundel (1380), Donnington (1393) and Ewelme (1437). These establishments had much in common with contemporary collegiate foundations. They were distinguished from the earlier foundations by having individual dwellings not exclusively under one roof; the chapel was also altogether distinct, although sometimes connected by a covered way. This provided a way of dispensing with the stricter monastic ideal without losing the benefit of communal life.

Loss of the monastic ideal had caused suspicion to fall upon the early infirmary-hall type of foundation. Benefactors and founders were attracted to the new smaller establishments which were easier to maintain, and throughout the later Middle Ages the maintenance and foundation of hospitals and almshouses became increasingly the provision of the laity. As merchants and tradesmen became more involved with the hospitals and almshouses they were more concerned to protect their investments. Consequently, their foundations were safeguarded with far greater secular control by the issue of strict regulations and frequent insistence that supervision of the foundation was overseen by nominees, often the mayor or members of a particular gild. This difference between the earlier and the later foundations is seen clearly by the success of the later hospitals and almshouses in surviving the Reformation. By contrast, many of the earliest foundations, strongly religious in character, were suppressed with the monasteries and gilds.

The story of the almshouses founded after 1350 is one of success. Founders ensured their buildings did not suffer from neglect by providing explicit instructions as to their governance. Detailed ordinances were drawn up which embodied a system of checks to guard against every threat to the continuance of the hospital's spiritual as well as eleemosynary work. Many hospitals of this date, including God's House, Ewelme, St John the Baptist and St John the Evangelist, Sherborne, and St Anthony's, York (1446) were incorporated upon foundation, ensuring their perpetual succession. Just what could occur if an institution was not properly incorporated is well illustrated by the sorry tale of St Cross Hospital, Winchester, in the years following the death of its refounder. Cardinal Beaufort (Bishop of Winchester 1404-47) paid considerable attention to his project at St Cross in the last five years of his life. It was no doubt intended as a lasting memorial to his long association with Winchester, but he failed to obtain the necessary charter of incorporation and within fifteen years of his death it fell victim to the power struggle of the Wars of the Roses and was robbed of most of the income intended for its support by Beaufort's 'unscrupulous' kinsfolk (Belfield 1982). By the time of Bishop Waynflete in 1485 the hospital, originally constituted for two chaplains, thirty-five brothers and three sisters, had been reduced to one priest and two brethren. Waynflete reported that 'in times past and by the craft of succeeding persons, the lordships, rents, tenements and possessions were wholly taken from the hospital and occupied by the power of noble persons' (Seymour 1947: 272).

Bishop Waynflete saved the buildings and the foundation of St Cross but the situation there was exceptional. Most of the later foundations survived without evident difficulty. They were generally smaller than the older hospitals, and a founder was usually able to endow his institution fully from its earliest days. Thus at Ewelme, in two grants of 1437 and 1442, William de la Pole, Duke of Suffolk, settled a sufficient endowment for the maintenance of two chaplains and thirteen poor men (*CPR 1436-41*: 80; *1441-46*: 54). Most of the institutions must have been adequately endowed, for there are remarkably few instances reported of decay or dilapidation of the fabric occurring at these foundations. It may well be that, as at Donnington, a sum was set aside 'to be put in a common coffer to treasure for the reparations of this our Almes House ...' (Money 1875-6: 264).

The statutes of Donnington reveal other ways in which the founder safeguarded his investment: 'Allsoe he hath ordained that the Minister every yeare betwixt the feast of St Michael and Christmas shall give his full accounts of all things he hath received and departed among his brethren and also spended in common profits before one of our Lord's Counsell which the Lord will assign in the presence of all the brethren of the Almes house gathered together ...' (Money 1875-6: 264). A similar provision for control and preservation of the foundation was made at Arundel where each year a written statement was to be rendered detailing the condition of the property with an inventory of the goods and chattels appended to the report.

As well as preserving the fabric of the building founders and patrons were also successful in preventing the neglect and abuses suffered by the older hospitals. Where abuses did occur it is significant that they were in foundations still under the control of, or manipulated by, the Crown. These foundations continued to be poorly administered and suffered abuses similar to those experienced at the earlier hospitals. For example, like St Cross Hospital, the foundation of William de la Pole's at Ewelme was another victim of political power struggles. Although William was executed as a traitor, the endowment was completed by his wife, Alice, in 1342 and the foundation was evidently well administered while the hospital remained within the family. But in the reign of Henry VIII the Suffolk estates in Ewelme were forfeited to the Crown on the attainder of the Earl of Lincoln, one of William's descendants, and became part of a royal manor. Nevertheless the foundation continued and survived the Dissolution. However, from the early seventeenth century Ewelme was used by the Crown as the recipient of a succession of corrodians which must have drained its revenues. Henry VII's foundation at Westminster was even less fortunate. Founded originally *c.* 1504 with the intention of providing board and lodging of a semi-communal nature for

> thirteen poor men, one an unbeneficed priest ... the houses should be kept in good repair as they are now and no payment for use ... (*SP Dom. 1547-65*: 537-8).

The ideal had clearly been departed from by 1563 when a petition of the almsmen revealed that

> wherein our predecessors enjoyed a hall where they kept a common table ... and had an attached garden for recreation ... about 16 years ago, Vincent, wardrobe of the beds to Henry VIII pretending

interest in the premises as of the gift of the king, granted the same to Nicholas Brigham who entered into the said hall, gardens and other premises and detained them during his life (*CClR 1500-09*: 146).

Whether or not the petitioners were re-established in the almshouse remains unknown.

The inmates at Westminster were menial servants of the king and one way to prevent abuses occurring was to control the recipients of the charity. While under the control of the Suffolk family, the inmates at Ewelme had been carefully selected in order to ensure further the preservation of their foundation with the Chancellor and Treasurer of England nominated as protectors. The Ewelme bedesmen were expected to be 'restful, peaceable, attending to prayer, reading and work' (*VCM Oxfordshire* 2: 97). The statutes of Arundel also laid down clear instructions as to admittance; the candidates were to be poor men, unmarried or widowers who from age, sickness or infirmity were unable to provide for their own sustenance and were selected by the master and majority of the existing brethren (Tierney 1834: 664-5). They were expected to be of good life and be able to repeat the Lord's Prayer, Salutation and Creed in Latin. Preference was given to tenants of the patron. At Arundel, the inmates were expected to be 'lettered or able at least to help the priest sing mass' (*VCH Sussex* 2: 97). At Westminster, and no doubt elsewhere, a copy of the ordinances was placed in the almshouse chapel, for it was still the task of every inmate to spend much of his time in prayer.

The new infirmary-hall type

The almshouses at Westminster had been founded in 1509 to 'pray for the king's good estate and afterwards his soul' (*CClR 1500-09*: 146). In 1438 the 'almessehouse' at Wells was described as

> lately erected in honour of Our Saviour, and the Virgin for the good estate of the King and the said bishop [Stafford] and their souls after death, for the souls of their parents and progenitors, of Nicholas Bubbewith, late bishop [founder], of the parents and benefactors of the present bishop and of all the faithful departed: also to maintain 24 poor persons in the same hospital to pray for the same estate and souls (*CPR 1436-41*: 187).

Benefactions for prayers did not decline dramatically before the Reformation and accordingly these new foundations were still much influenced by the concern of the founder for his soul. Thus the almspersons were not only the recipient of charity but had a charitable service to discharge. This ensured that the chapel retained its place of importance in the establishment and was often situated still adjoining the dwelling house, as it is at St Saviour's, Wells, separated from it by a carved oak screen (23).

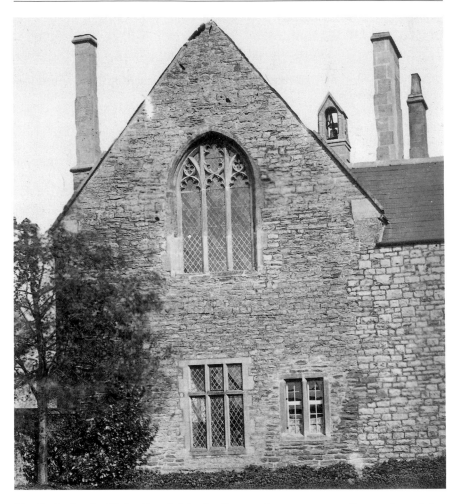

23 St Saviour's, Wells, founded in the fourteenth century, a smaller version of the infirmary-hall type hospital with chapel adjoining the dwelling house.

One of the finest surviving examples of this type of fifteenth-century almshouse, much of it in an almost complete state of preservation, is the hospital of St John the Baptist and St John the Evangelist at Sherborne (**24**). The exceptionally well-appointed chapel adjoins the east end of a two-storeyed infirmary hall, or dormitory, and extends the whole height of the building, enabling, in the long-established tradition of the infirmary-hall type of foundation, direct communication with both floors of the building. Nevertheless the domestic accommodation was separated from the chapel. The inmates could see the priest at the altar and share in divine service by means of a gallery on the upper floor and through an open-work screen below. The inmates were expected to say prayers five

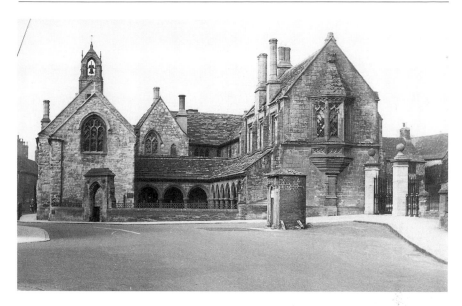

24 St John the Baptist and St John the Evangelist, Sherborne, founded 1437 in the tradition of the earlier hospitals.

times a day for the good estate of the founders and benefactors and to hear mass daily.

Because of its importance, the chapel was normally completed first, as it probably was at Sherborne in 1442 when 2s. 6d. was received towards the consecration of the altar by the bishop; other payments (2s. for wine, 6s. 8d. for the bishop and 3s. 4d. for an indulgence) were also made in connection with this event. The chapel contains its original south window (now restored), purchased at a cost of 8s. 4d., and an exceptionally fine late-fifteenth-century triptych (**25**).[1] The work at Sherborne was probably completed in 1448, the accounts of the foundation giving an interesting insight into the means of construction (Fowler 1951: 252-7).

The Sherborne accounts also reveal the financing of the project. The almshouse seems to have been a refoundation of an earlier institution which possibly occupied the same site. The earlier foundation was not wealthy — only £3 13s. 6d. was transferred to the new account when Henry VI issued his letters patent for incorporation on 11 July 1437 (*CPR 1436-41*: 77). There were no large-scale endowments to finance the building of the new almshouse but a house-to-house collection from the residents of Sherborne, raising £41 13s. 10d., formed the basis of the building fund. Additional benefactors and no less than five co-founders (Robert Neville, Bishop of Salisbury, Sir Humphrey Stafford, Margaret Goffe, John Fauntleroy and John Barrett) recorded in an early memorandum of the hospital, provided the remainder (Fowler 1951: 240-2).

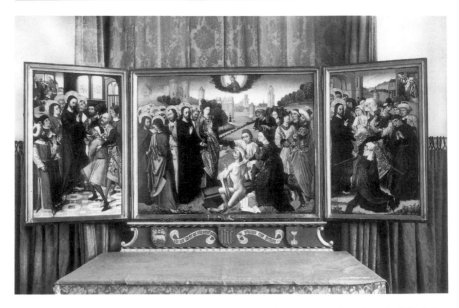

25 Exceptionally fine late fifteenth-century triptych equipping the chapel of St John the Baptist and St John the Evangelist, Sherborne.

With the possible exception of Robert Neville, the co-founders of Sherborne were not immensely wealthy magnates or clerics, and this may have limited the size of their foundation; the hall, measuring some 15 m by 6 m was considerably smaller than those of the early infirmary-hall type of hospital. The almshouse of St Saviour at Wells (**24**) was the largest of the new type of foundation, with a hall some 26 m long. However, an indenture for the building of the almshouse in 1436 shows a more traditional building ambition, stating that it should be erected on ground

> 160 feet long by ninety four feet [48.8 m by 38.7 m] wide at the west end and 114 feet [34.7 m] wide at the east end, consisting of one or more houses for twelve separate habitations ... (*PP1820*, 4: 346).

It would have been a very large structure for so few people, and in the event the completed building fell far short of the ideal.

Perhaps the founder of the hospital at Wells, Bishop Nicholas Bubbewith, ran short of funds. But more probably these new foundations were small from choice. Almost certainly Henry Chichele, Archbishop of Canterbury and founder of All Souls College, Oxford, could have established a larger foundation in his native town of Higham Ferrers should he have wished to do so.[2] The bedehouse there with its attached chapel remains a fine example of fifteenth-century architecture and obviously no expense was spared in its construction (**26**). But the hall measures only 19 m by 7 m

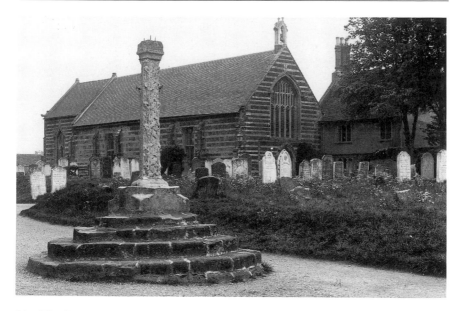

26 The Bede House at Higham Ferrers, the fifteenth century foundation of Henry Chichele, archbishop of Canterbury.

divided by wooden partitions. The numbers of inmates were limited (twelve bedesmen and a nurse). Thus the founder probably had the advantage of securing greater control over his institution, and with the increased number of regulations for the organization of the foundation the number of abuses could be reduced or even wiped out, ensuring the maintenance of the eleemosynary and more particularly the spiritual functions of the house.

The new model: the courtyard plan

The plans of foundations such as those at Higham Ferrers, Wells and Westminster were but a smaller model of the traditional style of infirmary hall and chapel with increased privacy. A marked break with tradition can be seen in the plans of another group of almshouses founded at the same time.

Most typically, these new almshouses took the form of a group of buildings surrounding a courtyard: a plan already familiar at contemporary manor-houses and collegiate establishments. One of the best-known examples is William de la Pole, Earl of Suffolk's foundation at Ewelme, set up in 1347 (**27**). De la Pole had been frequently resident at Donnington and was nominally the first master of the hospital there, probably overseeing the completion of the design of the founder Sir Richard Abberbury. De la Pole chose a similar plan for Ewelme − rows of individual dwellings

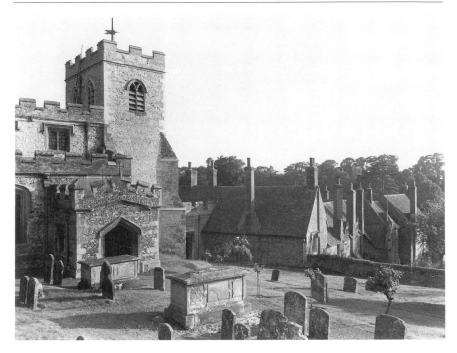

27 The hospital buildings, with church above, of William de la Pole's foundation at Ewelme, a fine example of the new fifteenth-century courtyard-plan foundations.

surrounding a courtyard and loosely connected to the church. Another notable foundation was at St Cross, where, by the middle of the fifteenth century Cardinal Beaufort had added his own expensive work of piety to the existing ancient hospital, choosing to erect an entirely new set of buildings around a quadrangle to the north-west of the church (**28**).

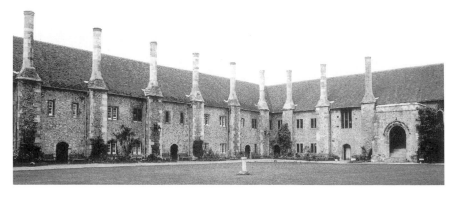

28 The almshouses of Noble Poverty, Cardinal Beaufort's fifteenth-century addition to the hospital of St Cross, Winchester with individual lodgings for the bedesmen.

For men like Cardinal Beaufort, who accumulated riches in the service of the Crown, or the newer men in service like the Fitzalans (Arundel) and the de la Poles (Ewelme) who made their fortune in the wars or in trade, one of the most obvious ways of perpetuating their memory or displaying their newly gained wealth was in the foundation of a hospital or almshouse. This also appealed to rich merchants like William Ford of Coventry. Ford's almshouses, founded *c.* 1509, are a spectacular work of piety. They comprise six timber-framed dwellings of two storeys arranged on the sides of a narrow courtyard, with hall and chapel at either end, entered from the street by a passage through the ground floor of the front range (**29**). Yet it is the even more magnificent façade which best demonstrates the handsome and most lavish nature of their construction (**30**). A range of oak uprights forms the constructional framing of the walls and each is decorated with a small pinnacled buttress. On the ground floor are nine single-light windows in three bays either side of the central doorway. But the main features are the three ranges of upper windows which project boldly from the wall, with richly carved barge-boards in the gables. Indeed, this front has been described as 'probably the most beautiful example of the English timbered house of the sixteenth century we possess' (Heath 1910: 82). Even now, after restoration, having been badly damaged during the Second World War, the almshouses provide a lasting memorial and tribute to their founder.

At Ford's hospital, it was the whole of the street front that was the object of conspicuous display. More usually, particularly in the monastic and collegiate establishments, it was the gatehouse that was the focus of attention. St Giles Hospital, Kepier, Durham (**10**), had already been provided with its fine gatehouse *c.* 1314, and the newer courtyard plans gave an obvious opportunity for such an embellishment. The gatehouse is the sole survivor of the domestic buildings of the small foundation of Abbot Bere at Glastonbury, ornamented on its exterior with the arms of Henry VIII (**14**). One of the most striking of the surviving gatehouses is that of St Cross, Winchester (**31**). Dating to the mid-fifteenth century it stands as a truly monumental structure of three storeys. The exterior face bears a frieze of heads and niches one of which contains a kneeling effigy of the founder, Cardinal Beaufort, and in the spandrels are the royal arms of England and the arms of the founder. The interior face is similarly embellished, although the features are less ornate and there is an octagonal stair-turret which rises higher than the building itself. Even in the name of the gatehouse, the Beaufort Tower, the cardinal's remembrance on earth had been assured.

The desire to preserve one's name was not the only reason which prompted the foundation of these establishments. In large part, they were still inspired by a memorial purpose and were the focus of the same charitable aspirations as was the new infirmary-hall type of foundation. Many embodied what were, to all intents, provision for a chantry in their

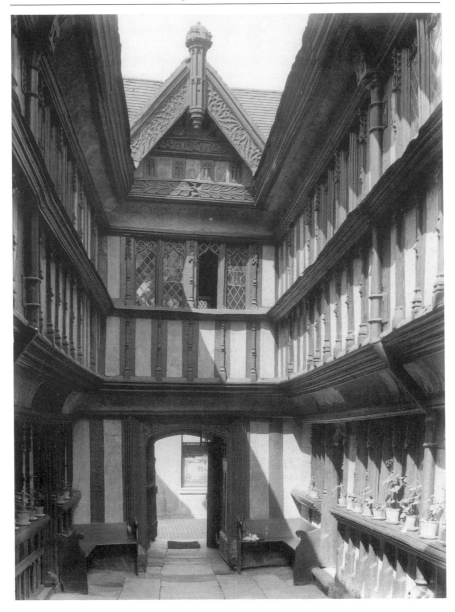

29 Individual dwellings surrounding a small courtyard of William Ford's almshouses at Coventry, *c.* 1509.

constitution, as at Donnington, where the statutes ordered the thirteen poor men.

> to pray for the state of Sir Richard Abberbury, his sonne and Alice his wife, and for all his heyres that live and for the soules of Sir

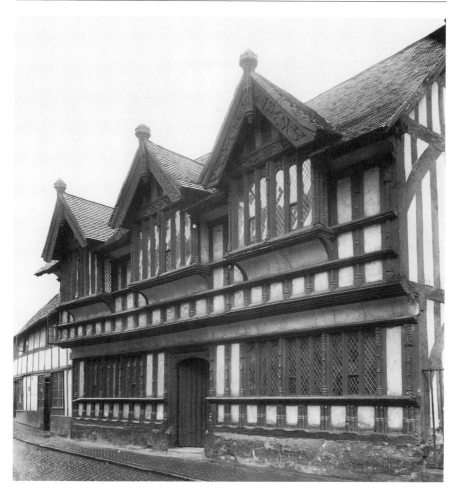

30 The façade of Ford's almshouses, Coventry, badly damaged in the Second World War but restored to their original beauty.

> Richard Abberbury, knight, our founder and Anne his wife and all his children that be dead and for the soules that he is due and in debt to pray for and for all Christians (Money 1875-6: 265).

In the statutes of Ewelme provision is also made for 'prayoure in which we grete trust and hope to our grete relief and increase of our merite and joy finally' (Clay 1909: 88). Indeed, the inmates at Ewelme were kept at almost constant prayer; private prayer at their bedside was followed by matins and prime soon after six, they attended mass at nine, bedes at two, evensong and compline at three and at about six the final bidding prayer was said around the founder's tomb. So important was this round of prayer considered to be that attendance at the divine offices was to be

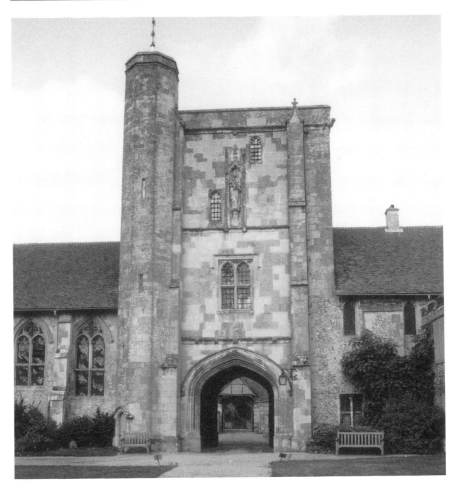

31 Gatehouse of St Cross, Winchester.

strictly observed and latecomers were subject to a fine of 1d. or 2d. out of
their weekly allowance of 1s. 2d.

At Ewelme and St Cross, the chapel was detached from
the dwellings, a distinguishing characteristic of these foundations. At
Donnington there was no special chapel, but the inmates and priest were
enjoined to 'goe everyday to heare Masses among the ffreers [friars] ...'
(Money 1875-6: 265). The friars' church at Donnington was adjacent to
the almshouse and would have been more convenient than the parish
church which was 0.8 km distant.

At Ewelme the almshouses were built adjoining the parish church of St
Mary, linked by the tower which had two low doorways on the ground
floor in each side wall in order that processions might make a complete

circuit of the exterior of the church when required. The church had been built by William de la Pole a few years prior to his founding of the almshouse. To make provision for his bedesmen, he added an aisle to the south of the chancel for use as the hospital chapel dedicated to St John the Baptist. The chapel was of considerable size, as wide as the chancel and of the same length. It is the most ornamental part of the building, its special feature being a richly panelled roof of oak. Leland, in the time of Henry VIII, recorded an inscription on the walls 'Pray for the soules of John, Duke of Suffolk and Elizabeth his wife' (Cook 1947: 177). John, son of William de la Pole and his wife Alice, was probably responsible for the magnificent alabaster tomb of Alice, Duchess of Suffolk, which, surmounted by a stone canopy, stands within an opening dividing the chapel of St John the Baptist from the chancel (32).

The use of an existing ecclesiastical institution, as at Donnington and Ewelme, was not uncommon in foundations of this date. No better example may be found than at the Hosier almshouses at Ludlow, founded in 1482 by John Hosier, a Ludlow draper, who attached his charity to the long-established Palmers' Gild. The gild had already endowed its own chapel situated in the north chancel chapel of the nearby church of St Lawrence, and the inmates of the almshouse were able to use the very fine gild chapel at no extra cost to the charity. A similar provision was made for use of the church of St Helen by the bedesmen of the 'Feat' or Long Alley almshouses at Abingdon. A close connection existed between the church and the Gild of the Holy Cross, the founders of the almshouse, with the gild adding a fourth aisle to the church in the fifteenth century (Preston 1929: 18-20).

Elsewhere completely new chapels were built. A small perpendicular chapel survives from Abbot Bere's foundation at Glastonbury (later known as St Patrick's), situated just outside the precincts of the abbey. A hospital existed on the site as early as 1246 but was rebuilt by Abbot Bere *c.* 1512 with a new chapel always totally separate from the domestic buildings. Within the chapel is preserved the altar from the original foundation.

Occasionally the new traditions were mixed with the old, as at Forster's foundation in Bristol of *c.* 1484. The almshouses originally consisted of thirteen separate chambers on two storeys, with the chapel still adjoining although quite distinct from the dwellings. The chapel was built 'In honour of God to the Three Kings of Cologne' (Jordan 1960: 26b) and, small though it is, is as fine as any of the chapels of the earlier hospitals.

The dwellings

The dwellings of the new infirmary-hall type of foundation, with their cubicles, were probably very similar to those of the later remodelled halls of the early hospitals. Privacy was considered important enough for foundations deeds, like that of Sherborne of 1437-8, to ordain that

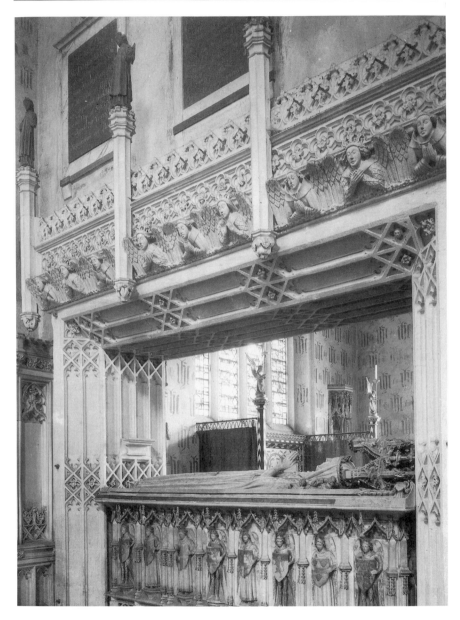

32 The alabaster tomb of Alice Duchess of Suffolk, wife of William de la Pole, placed in his hospital chapel of St John the Baptist, Ewelme.

every one of the saide Sixteyne pore men and wymmen . . . shall haue always . . . a bedde and a bedde place by him selfe . . . and that the men could sleep at night by themself, and that there be a reasonable and sufficient clusure by twixt them (Fowler 1951: 256-7).

Just how large this was is not prescribed but the 3.0 by 2.4 m of the cubicles at Stamford and Wells was probably considered adequate.

At St Saviour's, Wells, there may also have been some discrimination among places, very much akin to that practised in some of the older foundations. St Saviour's was intended for the relief of the burgessess of the city — for twelve poor tenants of the Dean and Chapter and of the Bishop of Bath and Wells and others of the parish of St Cuthbert (the parish in which the almshouse is sited), and for twelve other poor burgesses unable to live except by begging. To the burgesses nominated by the bishop were assigned the more 'honourable places' (Parker 1866: 50-63).

The separate apartments may have been considered an improvement on the conditions prevailing in the earliest hospitals, but many of them must still have been cold and gloomy. The north-west view of the infirmary hall at Higham Ferrers (26) shows only two small windows in the side wall and at the same institution there was, as yet, only a single fireplace situated in the south wall which was made up every morning before the men arose and set with water and a dish for washing. Single fireplaces were apparently quite common, also existing at Stamford and Wells. At Sherborne fires were permitted in the women's lodgings in the winter, presumably in addition to the single fire of the men's dormitory.

The cubicles at Higham Ferrers still retain some of the inmates' lockers, suggesting an increased emphasis on the holding of private property by this date. And these foundations did provide more for those in reduced circumstances than for those suffering absolute poverty. The inmates of Higham Ferrers were certainly not paupers. Each brother was expected to bring, on admittance: a bedstead, a mattress, bolster, pillow, two pairs of sheets, blanket, coverlet, brass pot of two gallons, a brass pan, and pewter dish and saucer. If he possessed no suitable gown he could have the best gown of his deceased predecessor for which he should pay 3s. 4d. together with 4d. for the brethren to make merry, 6d. for oatmeal and salt, 2d. to the bedmaker and 1d. to the barber (*VCH Northamptonshire* 2: 178-9). At Sherborne it was the *householders* of the town who were to be preferred above all others; at Wells it was the reduced *burgesses*, and Cardinal Beaufort's refoundation at St Cross was to consist of gentlefolk who could no longer support themselves or former members of the cardinal's household.

It was obvious that the inmates of these hospitals could not be bound to total poverty. At Westminster and Ewelme a man could possess property worth up to £4 a year before he had to leave the almshouse. By 1478 the inmates of St Nicholas's Hospital, Salisbury, were expected to enter with property of which the master was ordered to take charge and see that their clothes and other necessaries were provided from it.

Cardinal Beaufort's refoundation at St Cross was appropriately named the 'House of Noble Poverty', and for such a class of inmate the standards of comfort increased significantly. As with the other courtyard plan foundations of this date, the emphasis was on the total separation of the dwellings from the hall, along with improvements in comfort. What especially distinguished these foundations was that each dwelling became a distinct unit with its own entrance. The founder's intention at Ewelme, as expressed in the statutes, was specifically that

> the minister ... and pore men have and holde a certeyn place by themself within the said house of almesse, that is to saying a lityle house, a celle or a chamber with a chimney and other necessarys in the same (Clay 1909: 120)

At Ewelme this arrangement can still be seen. The rooms of the inmates are quite separate, consisting of a sitting-room on the ground floor and a bedroom over. A covered way or cloister, protecting the dwellings and forming a passage to the church, extends all around the quadrangle.

The importance of this privacy is stressed in the precise instructions left by founders as to the construction of their foundations. The clearest surviving set of instructions comes from Ralph, Lord Cromwell's foundation at Tattershall, built some years after his death in 1485/6. Fulfilling the wishes of the founder, a building agreement for the construction of the almshouse shows obvious concern for the well-being of the inmates. An existing older building was to be demolished and its timbers reused to construct a range 52.4 m in length and 5.8 m across. Within this range, which was to be built adjoining the churchyard, each of the thirteen bedesmen was to have his private chamber 'every chamber of the same thirteen chambers to have two windows, either window to be of two lights of a competent height' (Salzman 1967: 544-5).

Along with the increased emphasis on privacy, personal living standards also rose. This is particularly noticeable in the provision of garderobes and chimneys. St Cross gives exceptionally fine examples of the provision of both these amenities (**28, 33**). A garderobe was constructed with each dwelling. These are visible externally, situated to the rear of the range in pairs, marked by a series of gabled projections over a watercourse diverted from the nearby river Itchen. St Cross may have served as the model for Henry VII's almshouses at Westminster, built in the early sixteenth century. A ground plan shows that there, on the ground floor at least, each set of chambers had its own garderobe overhanging the Long Ditch.

Another major feature which greatly increased the comfort in these foundations was the provision of much improved heating. The almshouses at Westminster were, like St Cross, also provided with chimneys, a feature which was a prime requirement for these new foundations with their individual dwellings. Chimneys were also provided with the foundation at Ewelme, and each of the thirty-three chambers of John Hosier's almshouse at Ludlow (1486) was equipped with a fireplace. These chimneys were massive. At St Cross they form the main feature of the courtyard side of

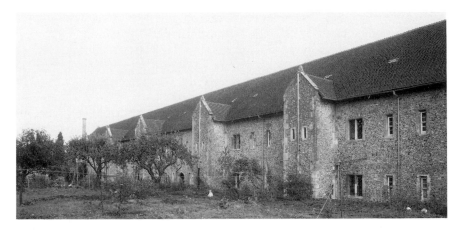

33 The rear of the almshouses St Cross, Winchester, showing the increased comfort of the fifteenth-century dwellings.

the range of dwellings with their fine projecting chimney-stacks with octagonal flue shafts and embattled coping, their very size and elaborate architectural detail indicating a great pride in their provision. Similarly it is the chimneys that attract attention as the most distinctive architectural feature of the hospital of St John the Baptist, Lichfield, founded *c.* 1140 and rebuilt on refoundation in 1495. The main east range of the hospital fronts on to St John Street and it is on the range facing the street that eight massive chimney-stacks of red brick, projecting some distance from the face of the wall, were constructed (**21**).

The hall

The provision of chimneys and individual chambers was indicative of a changing way of life. But almost all these new foundations were still provided with a hall of some size and standing. However, the function of the hall was also beginning to change. Increasingly used principally as a centre for social gatherings, both private and public, the fifteenth-century hall became the focus of public display in the new almshouse complexes.

The Gild of St Anthony, as founder of the almshouse of St Anthony's, York, founded in 1446, also used the hall as a meeting place and for such a purpose ensured that it was a showpiece (**34**). Much of the original mid-fifteenth-century hall remains and it is a splendid example of the domestic architecture of that date. Originally comprising a first-floor aisled hall with tie-beam roof, it was extended towards the east at the end of the fifteenth century, adding another six bays. New aisles were also built, incorporating the rooms on either side of the hall, and the whole was reroofed. The screens passage was at the east end, with a fine minstrels' gallery over.

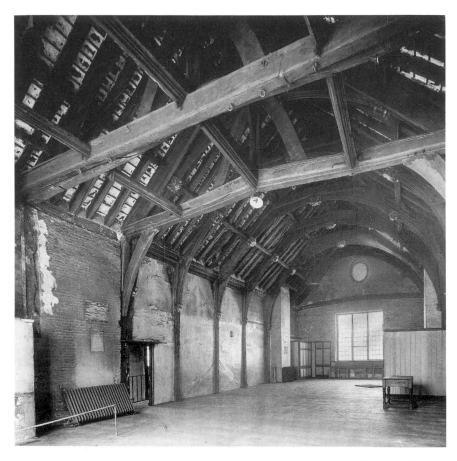

34 By the fifteenth century, expectations of comfort were high as shown at St Anthony's Hall, York built by the Gild of St Anthony's and shared with the almshouses founded by the gild in 1446.

A very similar design was selected for the very fine 'Brethren's Hall' at Cardinal Beaufort's new foundation of St Cross (**35**). In keeping with the other buildings of the hospital, little expense would have been spared in the construction and fitting out of the hall. Adjoining the gatehouse to the west, the hall forms the centre of the western range and is still very much as it would have appeared in the fifteenth century, 12.2 m in length, 7.3 m wide and 9.8 m high. At the east end is the slightly raised dais. The screens passage and gallery are positioned at the west end. The chief feature of the room is its fine timbered roof of four bays, with an opening to allow the smoke to escape from the still visible central hearth.

All meals were still supposed to be taken in these halls. Regulations, although far fewer, continued to order inmates to dine together. In 1442, at the hospital of the Holy Cross, Stratford-upon-Avon, the brethren were

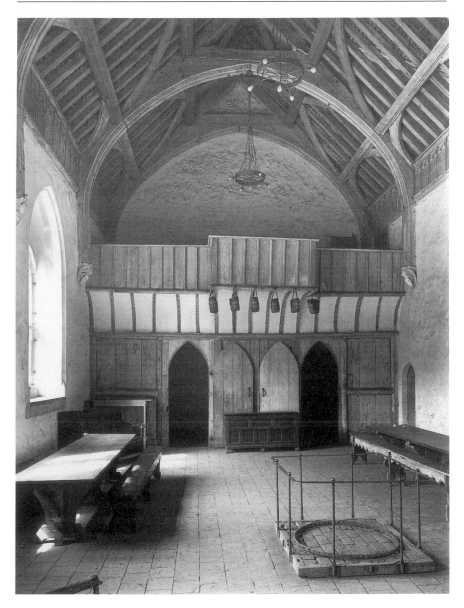

35 The Brethren's Hall at St Cross, Winchester, shows a domestic building that not only served to fulfil the communal element still required at this date but also illustrates the high standards and increased comfort to be found in these foundations.

required to eat and drink together in one house, although they were allowed to sleep at night in their own chambers (Westlake 1919: 113). Nevertheless, there were signs of change. The tendency was increasing for the substitution of daily meals as a dole in the form of cash. The brethren at the bedehouse of Higham Ferrers were given 7d. a week to buy their victuals. Each brother was to buy his meat on Saturday and bring it to the woman (nurse), telling her what portion she should cook for the morrow and the remainder she was to 'powder up' against Wednesday. On Sunday she was to set on the pot and make them a good pottage, giving each man his own dish and saving the rest for Monday's dinner. On Wednesday she was to set on the pot as for Sunday (*VCH Northamptonshire* 2: 178-9).

The brethren at Higham Ferrers were beginning to gain a little independence and choice in their actions. An alternative method of self-provision had been favoured at St Bartholomew's, Sandwich, at the beginning of the fourteenth century. Here every day a quantity of porridge, beans, peas or other vegetables was prepared in the kitchen, for common use. Every person was to put his or her meat into the pot, and the cook returned it when sufficiently boiled with a basin of porridge. No one was permitted to use a separate pot on the common fire, as it was the only fire in the hospital. The brethren were provided with their victuals but were also allowed 2d. a week for beer (Boys 1792: 18-19).

Money payments in lieu of food allowances were becoming more common in the fifteenth century but the departure from the idea of a communal life within a caring environment was far from complete. Inmates still received many of the traditional services found in the early hospitals. In 1534 the inmates of Higham Ferrers were still receiving 7d. per week each, but in addition they were given five yards (4.6 m) of cloth at Christmas, eight loads of firewood per annum, 10s. at Easter for wood, 5s. per annum for shaving (a barber attended every Friday) and 5s. per annum to maintain the lamp in their dormitory (*L & P Henry VIII* 18(1): 283). For as long as so much continued to be provided for the inmates in the long-established manner, the more traditional set of buildings would still be required.

Masters and their residences

One set of buildings that had definitely decreased in scale was accommodation for resident staff. With the increased purchase of many items and corresponding decrease in the size of the establishment and numbers of inmates, there was less need for the maintenance of the large bodies of staff that characterized the early foundations. Of the post-1350 foundations, only at Browne's Hospital, Stamford, is there any evidence of a large complex of domestic buildings after the manner of a monastic-type precinct (36).

Even at Stamford, however, the sick were cared for by the other female inmates who shared a room. As they already occupied a dwelling within the hospital, no special buildings were needed for their shelter. Likewise the woman 'attendant' at Higham Ferrers occupied one of the cubicles. At Sherborne, the foundation deed provided for a woman to be engaged to prepare the meals of the inmates, to wash and 'wring' for the sixteen poor

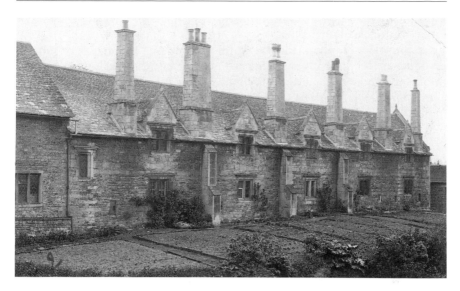

36 Browne's Hospital, Stamford, a fourteenth-century almshouse, unusually for that date, founded with small, but complete monastic-type complex.

feeble men and women, to make their beds and other things in the house as would a housewife (Fowler 1951: 242). She was evidently allotted a special apartment, payment being recorded in 1451-2 of 16d. for timber to repair the 'huswyves chamber', probably situated with the other women's dwellings on the upper floor of the new infirmary hall (Mayo 1926: 46-8). In 1483-4, also at Sherborne, a matron first appears in the accounts, and she was later provided with a woman to help her (Fowler 1951: 248-9).

The spiritual needs of the inmates were also served by fewer staff; at most, one or two chaplains. At Wells, the sole chaplain also provided the poor with their daily meal. Again no special building was required as the chaplain resided in a 'certain chamber on the western side of the hospital' (Parker 1866: 61). A single room was also set aside for the chaplain at Sherborne; payment is entered into the account of 1455-6 for a man 'making divers necessary repairs within the priests room', but it does not seem that he was always resident (Fowler 1951: 257).

Nevertheless, even if the numbers of staff were reduced there still had to be accommodation for the master. But the fine mansions of the masters of the earliest hospitals were not to be found, and indeed some of the strictest regulations of these later almshouses were concerned with the appointment and conduct of the master or warden. The abuses of absenteeism and pluralism, so rife in the early hospital foundations, were particularly attacked. Obligations to reside occur in almost all the statutes of this date. One such example comes from Arundel where the master was ordered 'to reside constantly within the walls of the hospital, to superintend the conduct and promote the comfort of the community' (Seymour 1947:

272). The master at Arundel probably occupied rooms in the western range of the quadrangle.

At Browne's Hospital, Stamford, the master was forbidden 'to mix up his office or service with any other benefice or ecclesiastical office or farm or other promotion whatever whereupon he shall be able to live comfortable' (Seymour 1947: 122). His lodgings were probably in two chambers on the upper floor of the enclosed court to the north of the traditionally placed hall and chapel. The chapel continued through two storeys, and when not in attendance the warden had a direct view to the chapel through a squint in an upper-floor chamber.

The master at Ewelme was granted the concession of holding one other benefice, but this was made dependent upon his continued residence within the hospital. William de la Pole attempted to attract a high calibre of master, if possible from the University of Oxford. The priest would have occupied the choicest part of the site – on the first floor flanking the church on the east, in an excellent position to overlook the activities of the inmates.

No doubt all the masters' residences were in the choicest part of the site, as they most certainly were at St Cross where the master occupied rooms over the porter's lodge and within the dominating Beaufort Tower. In the early seventeenth century, part of the western range was also appropriated for his use. Even at the small almshouse at Walthamstow, founded by George Monoux *c.* 1515, the master occupied a very pleasant situation in the attractive gabled lodging that formed the centre of the main building.

But progressively the need for a specially appointed master declined. Almsfolk began to take more responsibility for their foundations upon themselves. Much of the organization came to be provided by the inmates. At Higham Ferrers, the senior bedesman was termed the prior; no master was deemed necessary. A prior was also elected from among the sixteen poor at Sherborne and he was to have rule and governance in the absence of the master. The foundation at Sherborne was also governed by twenty brethren who seemed to form a 'Fraternity of the House', in existence as a religious gild. In 1446-7 the master refers to himself as 'master of the Gild of the almshouse' and in 1476-7 a new master, John Brance, with Margaret his wife, gave £5 to be admitted as participators in the prayers of the Brotherhood of the Almshouses, it soon becoming customary to make a donation of £5 at the time of taking office (Fowler, 1951: 245). These brethren were unlikely to have been resident, and this form of government may well have existed elsewhere.

Postscript: the Savoy

At the height of the foundation movement in favour of new, smaller hospitals with individual dwellings, was built the Savoy Hospital, London

(1505-17), an infirmary hall in the traditional manner of vast proportions. With the construction of the Savoy, the apogee of the infirmary-hall design was reached. The hospital was founded by Henry VII and building was under way by the time of his death in 1509. His design, known from plans and surveys of the seventeenth and eighteenth centuries, was completed in 1517. The main structure was cruciform with a great 'nave' of twelve bays and terminating chapel, forming an overall length of 96.3 m. The 'transepts' were over 61 m from north to south and, like the hall, were only 9.1 m wide; this proportion of width compared to length being typical of the early infirmary-hall type of plan.

This vast structure was essentially a dormitory to provide, in the words of the king's will, 'oon hundreth bedds' (Colvin 1975: 198). The easternmost part of the dormitory contained the Lady Chapel, while the northern end of the north transept was partitioned off to form St Katherine's chapel. Thus, in long-established tradition, every bed was in sight of an altar. Also in traditional manner, those admitted were to go first to the chapel and offer a prayer for the founder and thence to the dormitory where the beds were allotted to them by the matrons and sisters.

But the Savoy was not an anachronism. It was built for a special purpose, the provision of temporary relief 'garnished to receive and lodge nightly oon hundreth pouer folks' (Colvin 1975: 198). Only one night's food and lodging was provided, except for the sick who remained and received medical care and attention. This care began with the ritual undertaken on admittance by the provision of hot baths, delousing ovens for clothes and fresh gowns emblazoned with the Tudor livery to give no doubt as to the identity of the benefactor. In addition, and more significantly, two permanent physicians, 'honest men' skilled in medicine and surgery, were permanently employed whose duty it was to visit the sick mornings and afternoons when necessary (Bullough 1961: 74-7). Physicians and surgeons had been visitors or wardens of hospitals from early times but it is possible that, from the end of the thirteenth century, many of the early physicians disappeared from the hospitals, particularly those following a religious rule. This was due to papal regulations restricting the practice and study of medicine by men of the church. Physicians make a reappearance in the hospital records in the late fourteenth century but they were mainly absentees such as Simon Bredon, who was nominally warden of the Newark Hospital in Maidstone, but from 1358 was also physician to Joanna, Queen of Scots. The smaller hospitals of the later Middle Ages did not have the resources to finance permanent medical staff and were simply not built to a scale to warrant such a provision. By providing patients with the regular attendance of physicians and surgeons the Savoy may be seen not as the last of the ancient infirmary-hall foundations but the first of the 'modern' hospitals.

CHAPTER FIVE

POST-REFORMATION CHANGES

The foundation of hospitals and almshouses had been slowing since *c.* 1480 and practically ceased in the decades immediately following the Reformation.[1] Yet in the mid sixteenth century there was a desperate need for accommodation of this kind. The problem had been recognized as early as 1509 by Henry VII when he stated that

> there be few or noon such commune Hospitalls within this our Realme, and that for lack of them, infinite nombre of pouer needie people miserable dailly die, no man putting hande of helpe or remedie (Clay 1909: 12).

The problem was exacerbated by the numbers evicted from the hospitals and monastic houses and by 1550 the extensive work of providing accommodation for the poor carried out by the religious houses and pre-Reformation hospitals had been much diminished by the dissolution of many of these institutions. This was recognized in the *Supplication of the Poore Commons* (1546) about the plight of 'poor impotent creatures' who

> . . . then had hospitals and almshouses to be lodged in, but noew they lye and strewene in the stretes. Then was their number great, but now much greater (Clay 1909: 226).

In London, for example, which possessed about thirty-four hospitals and almshouses during the Middle Ages, most of which followed the Augustinian rule, the number of institutions was greatly reduced. Refuges were urgently needed for the

> ayde and comforte of the poore, sykke, blynde, aged and impotent persones, beying not hable to help theymselffs (Rawcliffe 1984: 17).

In the years following the Reformation there was certainly an increase in the problem of poverty. The mid sixteenth century saw a marked increase in population and ever-rising inflation. Debasement of the coinage and the continued rise in rents and prices forced many into difficulties. Furthermore, after 1541 the number and amount of benefactors for all religious purposes, including the relief of the poor, had declined appreciably.

With the demise of the monastic houses, there had to be a significant change in the distribution of charitable interests. Many patrons who had previously given to the religious now focused their attention on the poor. Prices stabilized *c.* 1560 and from that date the total number of gifts to the poor rose dramatically. Most importantly, almost half this amount was specifically designated for the erection and endowment of almshouses. (For examples, especially in the rural counties, see Jordan 1959, *passim*.)

Some of these new foundations were large courtyard-plan hospitals, following in the tradition of the earlier hospitals of this type, founded by members of the nobility. These foundations made a significant contribution to the problem of housing the poor, yet in 1546 Stubbes could still report that

> there is a certain city in England called London where the poor lie in the street, upon pallets of straw, and well if they may have that too or else in the mire and dirt as commonly is seen, having neither house to put in their heads nor covering to keep them from the cold nor yet to hide their shame (Stubbes 1595: 33).

It was not only in the towns that the problem of poverty was pressing. Many of the more modestly endowed almshouses fulfilled a need in the rural parishes. Their founders were much favoured in 1597 by the passing of an Act for the erecting of hospitals by which power was given to benefactors to give or bequeath lands in fee simple to erect a hospital or almshouses without the necessity of securing a special royal licence or Act of Parliament to achieve incorporation. This Act encouraged an outburst of building by men of lesser means, and with it the foundation of almshouses reached a new climax *c.* 1600 to be all but concluded by 1640.

With these foundations arose a new model for the almshouse consisting, typically, of a simple row of dwellings situated along a road close to the parish church with a small garden behind (**37**). These foundations were usually completely secular in their trusteeship and administration. But they continued to provide the improved standards of privacy and comfort of the better-off late medieval almshouses. Many were very small establishments, yet fulfilling a desperate need for this type of accommodation for the poor.

The fate of the early hospitals

Not only had the building of new hospitals and almshouses ceased after the Reformation, but many of the older foundations, particularly those associated with the monasteries and gilds which were chantry-like in their nature, were dissolved or tainted with suspicion. Some were extinguished with the lesser monasteries (1536), a few with the great houses (1539), and many more under the two Acts for the dissolution of the chantries

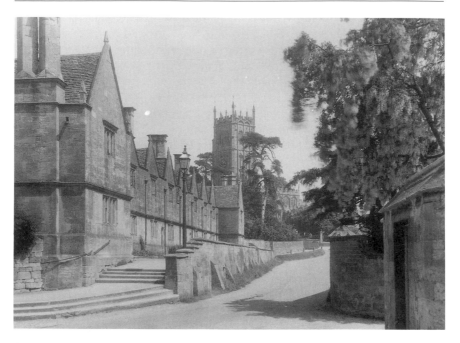

37   Baptist Hicks' foundation at Chipping Camden, typical of the new model of almshouse increasingly to be found from the sixteenth century.

(1545, 1547). By 1575 Archbishop Grindal felt obliged to write to the lord treasurer:

> the hospital ... is like to go to utter decay. ... For my own part I think often that those men which seek the spoil of hospitals ... did never read the 25th Chapter of Matthew, for if they did, and believed the same, how durst they give such advanture? And that if any hospitals be abused (as I think some are) it were a more Christian suit to seek Reformation than destruction (Clay 1909: 12).

In such an atmosphere not only were there no new foundations but building work in the surviving institutions was also halted. Few, if any, foundations can have felt secure at this time. There were, indeed, as many 'seeking the spoils of the hospitals' as there had been of the monasteries. St Nicholas Hospital, Salisbury, had been saved from dissolution largely due to the intervention of the earls of Pembroke but, nevertheless, struggled for over fifty years against the 'concealers' until saved by the efforts of the master Geoffrey Bigge (1593-1639). The hospital was finally granted a charter of refoundation by James I in 1610. Once secure in its future, with a new constitution for a master, chaplain and six poor and infirm, the hospital was able to embark upon a considerable rebuilding programme: a new kitchen was made for the hospital inmates, some of the old buildings were taken down and new rooms built, a second storey with four rooms was added over the former north chapel. In 1635, with the master now non-resident, and in keeping with contemporary trends, the chaplain's quarters were made more comfortable by the addition of a new study and private entrance and kitchen.

The Salisbury hospital had been well administered since the end of the fifteenth century, and was obviously in a good position to build for the future. But other institutions which survived dissolution were not so fortunate. Many had been suffering neglect from the mid fourteenth century, yet, in the face of urgent eleemosynary need, were crying out for 'reformation rather than destruction'. Among them was St Katherine's, Ledbury, under the patronage of the Dean and Chapter of Hereford 'which they had of late neglected'. In 1568 the hospital was described as 'at present concealed and converted to the uses of certain private men of sufficient wealth' (Morgan 1952: 88-132) and it was granted to John Scory, Bishop of Hereford (1559-86). However, Scory, having alienated the best estates in return for revenues scarcely half their value, was not the man under whom the hospital was likely to flourish and he was strongly opposed by the dean and chapter. It was not until 1580 that a decree restored the administration to the dean and chapter with instructions for stricter visitation and reformation of the charity. Once again an immediate building programme was begun, concentrating upon improving comfort for the inmates: the number of chimneys was increased, privies were added and a considerable amount of glazing undertaken.

Many of the older foundations were granted charters of refoundation. Once secure in their future, like St Nicholas, Salisbury, and St Katherine's, Ledbury, they began to improve their buildings very much as some foundations had already done in the years prior to the Reformation, by the addition of chimneys, garderobes and a proliferation of dwellings for use as private apartments. This resulted in a minor outburst of building work in these hospitals towards the end of the sixteenth century. After refoundation many came into the hands of the towns or corporations. Those hospitals which were already the property of the municipal authorities or which were ceded to them shortly after the Reformation, were among the first to be assured of their continuance. These foundations often attracted the support of the townsfolk and were the earliest to carry out rebuilding work.

Among this group was the hospital of St Giles, Norwich. The hospital had been well respected by the people of Norwich, supported by the mercantile aristocracy, and had been carefully administered throughout the fifteenth century. Nevertheless, Henry VIII had dissolved the foundation. After a petition, however, Edward VI conveyed the institution and all its endowments to the mayor and corporation free of all charges. The hospital was renamed Domus Dei; a lay master and a chaplain in residence were appointed to serve the inmates. In the next twenty years the hospital enjoyed the steady support of the citizens of Norwich, receiving numerous small bequests, and in 1572 Queen Elizabeth augmented the endowment. By the latter part of the sixteenth century, the hospital felt itself in a position to be able to undertake considerable alterations. The eastern chapel was also provided with a chimney in 1580 and another chamber was built over the Lady Chapel. An extra floor was inserted in both the infirmary hall and eastern chapel, at once doubling the numbers of poor able to be received and making provision for a schoolmaster and twelve children in 1581.

Another foundation which came into the hands of the municipal authorities was St Bartholomew's, Gloucester. Like St Katherine's, Ledbury, St Bartholomew's was in a poor state before the Reformation. Although not suppressed, the foundation continued to decline until early in the reign of Elizabeth when the inmates petitioned the queen that the hospital lacked necessary repairs, the church was ruinous, no services were held and in place of fifty-two inmates who formerly received 7d. weekly there were now only thirty-two receiving 4d. In 1564 the mayor and burgesses agreed to reform and to take control and financial responsibility for the hospital, and in 1569 the corporation records noted the building of nineteen new chambers (Ellis 1929: 203–6). These new chambers were built within the infirmary hall where excavations revealed considerable alterations dating to

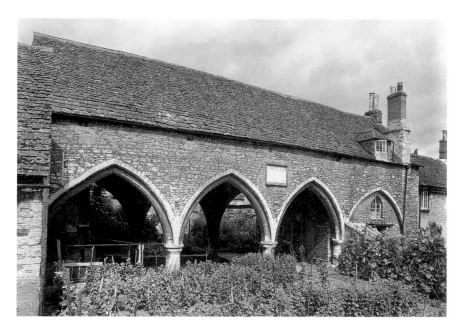

38 Arches of the infirmary hall of St John the Baptist, Cirencester remodelled, with the demand for privacy, into individual dwellings in the sixteenth century.

this period (Hurst 1974: 46). It was probably divided up in a manner similar to that of St John's Hospital, Cirencester, where the remains of six tenements incorporated within the arcades of the infirmary hall can still be identified (**38**).

The remodelling of the infirmary halls which took place at Norwich, Gloucester and Cirencester was a solution to rebuilding likely to have been favoured by many of the early hospitals. But in other foundations entirely separate buildings were constructed much akin to those of the new hospitals established in the fifteenth century (see Chapter IV). In 1558, Ralph Lamb of Winchester granted land to the mayor, bailiffs and commonalty of Winchester for the support of the poor of the hospital of St John the Baptist, founded sometime before 1270. His will detailed that this support should consist of maintenance for six poor and needy widows each to have a separate chamber with lock and key. These chambers were built in a court to the north of the existing infirmary hall. In 1572 'four separate mansions within the precincts' were constructed at the hospital of St Mary and St Thomas the Martyr at Ilford (*VCH Essex* 2: 187.19), and at God's House, Southampton, the old hospital buildings were almost completely demolished and replaced by an almshouse for eight persons between 1588 and 1593.

The post-Reformation courtyard-plan foundations

These new courtyard-plan foundations continued in the tradition of their counterparts of the later Middle Ages. Indeed, some of the new foundations were settled in earlier courtyard-plan buildings, used by the religious, which were then easily adapted to their use. Among them was the Earl of Leicester's foundation at Warwick which took over the premises of the combined gilds of the Holy Trinity and St George in 1571 (**39**). The gild buildings had been mostly rebuilt before the end of the fifteenth century. Originally entirely of timber-frame construction and set around four sides of a rectangular courtyard, the hospital was entered by a gatehouse in the south range (**40**). The buildings were admirably suited for a hospital in the traditional manner and required little alteration. The west range consisted of a long single-storeyed hall (two-storeyed at either end), open to the roof, and this building continued in use as a refectory for the hospital brethren. The northern part of the hall was partitioned off to provide extra rooms in the adjoining master's house. There is no evidence that special quarters were provided for the brethren. Some of the buildings had been allowed to decay but the dwellings of the gild chaplains, probably situated in the east range, would certainly have been available for use. The gildhall in the south range may also have been used to provide accommodation since it was divided into several compartments at a later date. Some building was carried out on conversion (the date 157 − was found during renovations in the 1950s), most notably consisting of the insertion of

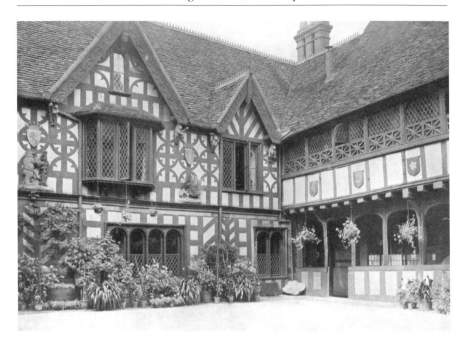

39 Benefactors like Robert Dudley, Earl of Leicester benefited from the Dissolution by taking over the premises of the combined gilds of Holy Trinity and St George at Warwick, making simple the conversion to a hospital.

numerous fireplaces, in 'outrageous' positions served by exterior chimneys – 'outrageous' on account of the flues having been carried out through walls enclosing timbers, and two fireplaces were actually placed with their chimneys standing on first-floor timbers (Pears 1966: 35-41).

More drastic reconstruction was required by Sir Thomas Coningsby for his hospital at Hereford (**41**). Founded by Sir Thomas in 1614, the buildings now form a quadrangle, the northern range of which preserves the hall and chapel dating to the thirteenth and fourteenth centuries, which belonged to the original owners of the site – the Knights of St John of Jerusalem. Coningsby added three ranges of twelve two-storeyed dwellings with the entrance from the street on the west and another gateway to a garden on the east. A gatehouse at the south end of the street front formerly led to Sir Thomas Coningsby's house, now a separate dwelling. Like Leicester's Hospital at Warwick, Coningsby's foundation, with its reused hall and chapel, had something in common with the early infirmary-hall type, yet with its individual dwellings also achieved the privacy and comforts of the courtyard plans of the fifteenth century.

Similar arrangements – a mixture of the old and new with local variations – were also evident in the newly built courtyard-plan foundations dating from the second half of the sixteenth century. A good example,

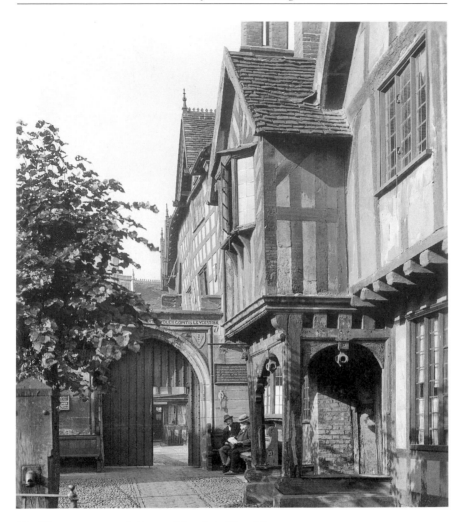

40 The entrance to Leicester Hospital, Warwick.

probably dating to the end of the century, is the hospital of St Mark at Audley End, built and endowed by the first Earl of Suffolk about the same time as he was building Audley End house (1603-16) (**42**). The plan consists of buildings grouped around two courtyards, each having ten dwellings, with the central range originally provided with a common hall and chapel adjoining at the east end.

Another interesting foundation, also dating from the end of the sixteenth century, is the Trinity Hospital at Croydon (1596-98) (**43**). Founded by John Whitgift, Archbishop of Canterbury, the hospital was described by Stow as 'a notable and memorable monument of our time' (Godfrey 1955: 57). The plan adopted here had more in common with the foundations at

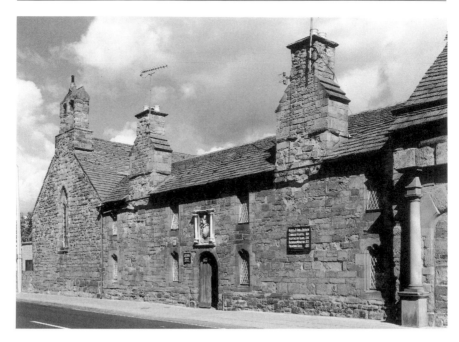

41　Sir Thomas Coningsby drastically reconstructed the buildings belonging to the Knights of St John to establish the Coningsby Hospital, Hereford, in 1614.

Ewelme and St Cross with a separate chapel and hall. The two-storeyed building of red brick forms a quadrangle entered from the street by a gatehouse. On either side of the gatehouse were the rooms of the almsfolk arranged in nine houses, entered by a door from the quadrangle, each containing four rooms, one for each inmate. Each room had a fireplace and a deep cupboard. The chapel, occupying the whole height of the

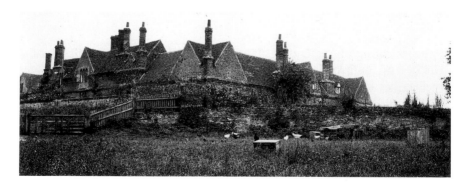

42　The College of St Mark, Audley End, one of the newly built courtyard-plan foundations which sprang up from the second half of the sixteenth century.

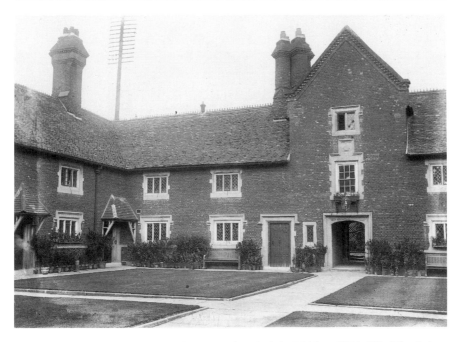

43 The impressive late sixteenth century hospital Archbishop Whitgift's Hospital, Croydon founded by Archbishop Whitgift.

building, is situated in the south-east corner of the easternmost range, which also contains the hall and kitchens.

Alongside the larger courtyard-plan hospitals were smaller versions of the same, founded by members of the gentry. Still standing today, although no longer used as such, is the small quadrangular almshouse known as Nappers Mite, situated in the centre of Dorchester, and built in 1615, under the provision of the will of the Dorset landowner, Sir Robert Napier, judge and Member of Parliament. Another example survives at Wotton-under-Edge, where the tiny courtyard of the almshouse founded by Hugh Perry (*c.* 1634), mercer and Sheriff of London, is almost filled by the contemporary chapel (**44**). Other establishments like the bedehouse at Newark (1556), Sir John Port's almshouses at Etwall (1556), and Sir Stephen Soames' foundation at Little Thurlow (1618) consisted of only three ranges around a courtyard.

The large courtyard plans as seen at Croydon and Audley End, and also to be found at Guildford (1619-22), Castle Rising (1609-15), Greenwich (1614) and elsewhere (Bray, 1627; Barnstaple, 1627; Long Melford, 1573), have been said to represent the post-Reformation evolution of the monastic ideal. But it was not the monastic spirit that prompted the building of these foundations. Whitgift's Hospital at Croydon, the 'notable and memorable monument' (Heath 1910: 102), was echoed and surpassed

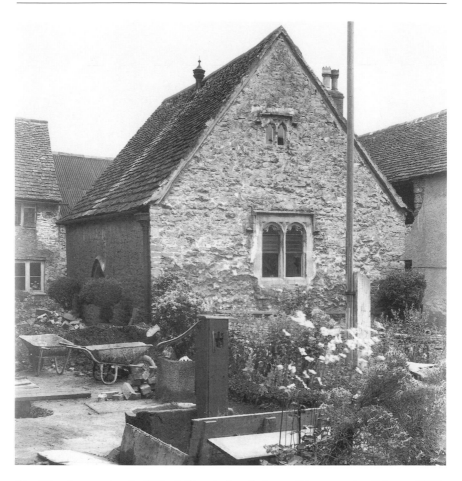

44   The tiny courtyard of Hugh Perry's foundation at Wotton-under-Edge, *c.* 1634, dominated by the chapel.

in a foundation of another archbishop of Canterbury, the Trinity Hospital at Guildford, founded by George Abbot in 1619-22. Practically identical in plan to the Trinity Hospital at Croydon, Abbot's hospital was considerably more ambitious in its architectural treatment. Situated in his native town where his father had been a cloth worker, the hospital was, for Abbot, a symbol of his success and as such is nothing short of a vehicle for self-conscious commemoration. Few would forget the huge gatehouse, facing on to the High Street, in the form of a three-storeyed tower of red brick consisting of a main central block flanked by two wings projecting on to the street line. At the angles of the tower are four octagonal turrets rising a stage above the tower (**45**). The architecture of the rest of the building was also of a sumptuous nature, particularly the fine brick chimney-stacks, with separate octagonal shafts and finely moulded caps and bases,

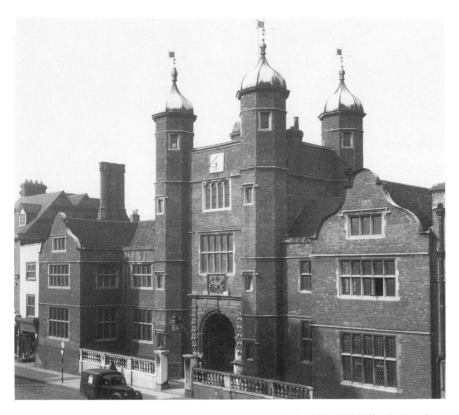

45 The monumental gatehouse of Abbot's Hospital, Guildford (1619), designed to rival the hospital at Croydon and perpetuate the memory of its founder.

still standing on the external walls of the brethren's lodgings. Abbot himself often occupied the fine set of rooms within the gatehouse which still contain some excellent early-seventeenth-century furniture (**46**). The chapel retains its original open-oak seating and there depicted, in the large stained-glass windows, are the personal arms of Abbot and those of the sees which he held.

No other better example of a personal monument can be found than Sir Thomas Coningsby's hospital at Hereford (1614). Although founded as a testimony of his gratitude to Providence for preserving him in his travels by land and sea as well as against malice at home, Sir Thomas ensured the Coningsby name would be remembered. The Coningsby monogram, TPC, abounds; in the chapel the stained-glass windows display the arms of the founder, while the walls are covered with various devices of the Coningsbys. Over the door leading from the chapel to the hall are two Ionic pillars framing a sculpture displaying the founder's arms, crest and mantling. Furthermore, the most senior inmate was to take the name of Coningsby and be called the Corporal of the Coningsby's Company of Old Servitors.

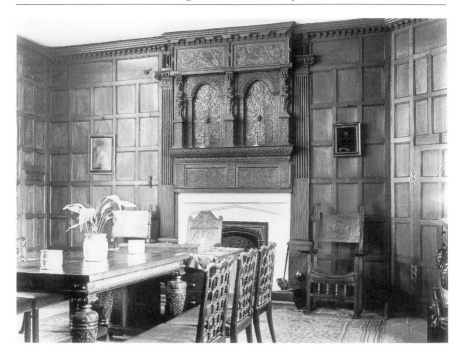

46 Archbishop Abbot's room in the gatehouse of his hospital at Guildford, designed for comfort and decorated with fine seventeenth-century pannelling.

Few could have attempted self-commemoration of the family on the scale of that of Henry Howard, Earl of Northampton. Between 1607 and his death in 1614 he had founded a large hospital of courtyard plan in the traditional manner at Greenwich (1614) and two smaller foundations at Castle Rising (1609) and Clun (1607). It is said that the earl built the hospitals as a lasting memorial to the various members of his family: at Greenwich in memory of his father whose death warrant was signed at Greenwich Palace; Castle Rising in remembrance of his grandfather, the third Duke of Norfolk, to whom Henry VIII had restored the castle shortly before his arrest and imprisonment; and Clun, said to be the most ancient family seat and favourite hunting ground of his brother. Whatever the reason, the earl certainly lavished great resources on these foundations, particularly the Trinity Hospital at Greenwich, the largest and most magnificent of his works. Now much modernized, it originally formed a spacious and well-planned set of buildings which had a cloistered walk around the courtyard with the unusual feature of an overshooting passage. In the centre of the sides were, to the east, the chapel which contains a kneeling effigy of the founder (47) and, to the west, a two-storeyed hall. Both hall and chapel projected from the main range of the building.

At Castle Rising, the hospital stands as originally planned and is a charming example of Norfolk brickwork. The dwellings, hall and chapel

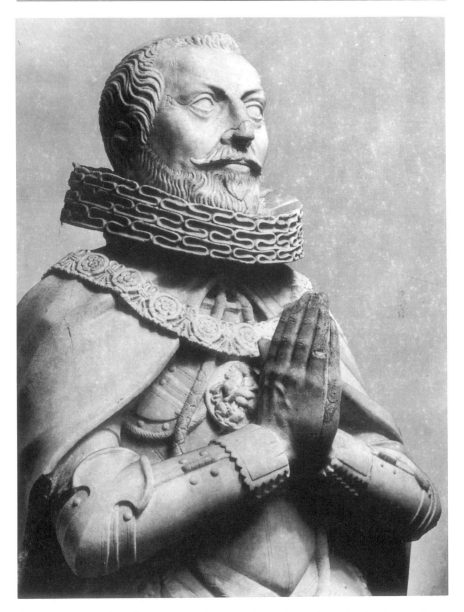

47 Detail from the effigy of Henry Howard, Earl of Northampton in the Trinity Hospital, Greenwich, founder of hospitals at Greenwich, Clun and Castle Rising established to commemorate various members of his family.

surround a courtyard and are single-storeyed except for the entrance way which is flanked on both sides by a small tower. The grander Sackville College, at East Grinstead, founded *c.* 1616 by the second Earl of Dorset, is almost identical in plan − another beautiful quadrangle built entirely of

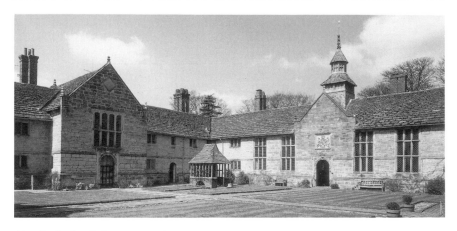

48   Sackville College, East Grinstead, a typical quadrangular plan of the early sixteenth century.

sandstone (**48**) and still retaining an impressive hall (**49**). Henry Howard's earliest foundation, the Trinity Hospital at Clun, though more modest in plan, is none the less an imposing building in the small town, with a fine group of three stepped central dormers on the south façade.

Maintenance of the post-Reformation foundations

Such costly investments warranted careful supervision to maintain the purpose of the foundation and to keep the buildings in good order. The founders of these large courtyard-plan hospitals usually ensured the incorporation of their foundation from an early date. Failure to incorporate was likely to lead to difficulty, as it did at the Sackville Hospital at East Grinstead. The start of building was considerably delayed after the death of the founder Robert Sackville, second Earl of Dorset, in 1609. Robert had bequeathed £1,000 for the foundation but many of the Sackville lands were alienated by the third Earl of Dorset with the purchasers refusing to acknowledge liability for the college; consequently the charter of incorporation was delayed until 1631. But for the most part, these institutions were well endowed and administered and there are remarkably few instances of decay, dilapidation or complaints of maladministration in the larger post-Reformation hospitals.

There was not only a need for careful planning to ensure the future of a foundation but once in existence there was certainly an urgent need for strict control. No doubt aware of former abuses and the problems arising from royal control of the foundations as seen at Westminster and Ewelme, the new hospitals drew up statutes and regulations in great detail. The task was often carried out by fellow members of the family or others in the peer group: the Earl of Suffolk and five others laid down the rules for

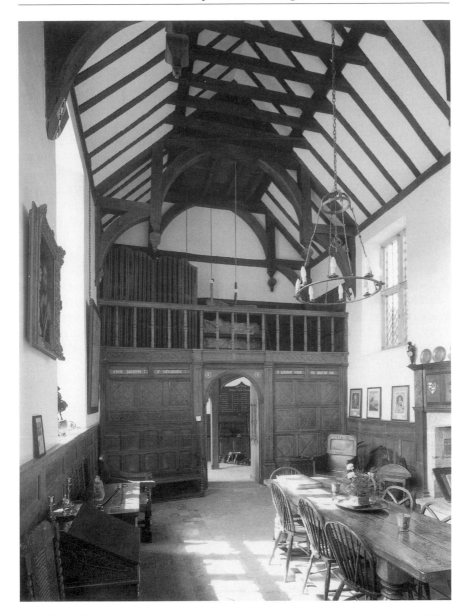

49 The hall, Sackville College, East Grinstead showing the remaining vestiges of the once totally communal living.

Clun, and the earls of Arundel and their heirs performed a similar task for the Trinity Hospital, Greenwich. Elaborate provision was made for visitation, and strict rules were laid down for the appointment of the warden or, as at Castle Rising, the governess. The warden was frequently expected to be 'able to read and write perfectly and to cost accounts, to be single and at least 40' (Clun), and was to be resident having

> all the rooms below stairs between the chapel and the gate, and private use for himself of the common hall and kitchen at all times of the year except when stated on festival days (*PP 1837-8* 26: 706-10).

Further rules were laid down as to the character of the inmates to ensure no blemish would arise to smear the good name of the foundations. The inmates were never selected from the absolutely poor, although they were not allowed to possess a great deal of property – no more than an income of £5 at Warwick or land worth 20s. or goods exceeding twenty marks at Greenwich. They were also expected to have a certain income. For example the bedesmen of Clun were required to enter into bond the sum of £10 to the bailiff of Bishops Castle before being allowed entry into the hospital. The inmates were very often tenants or servants selected from the estates of the founder as at Leicester's Hospital, Warwick, where preference was given to those wounded in the war and those decayed by misfortune rather than 'wicked wastefulness and notorious consuming' (*PP 1837-8* 26: 767). At Greenwich too, it was carefully stipulated that the inmates were to be 'decayed by casual means and not through a dissolute life' (*PP 1834* 22: 5-18).

The new model of almshouse

The inmates of the post-Reformation foundations expected higher standards and this gave rise to the development of spacious courtyard-plan hospitals which allowed considerable comfort and privacy for their inmates. In comparison with the early infirmary-hall type of design they provided for relatively few inmates – twenty at Greenwich, thirteen at Castle Rising, thirteen at Clun and equally small numbers elsewhere. Some, like Greenwich, were still pre-Reformation in character, providing for almost total maintenance of their almsfolk, where a butler, cook and poor woman attended upon the inmates who were also provided with the services of a laundress and barber. Provision for staff still took up a considerable amount of space in this establishment. Others, like Clun, provided individually for their inmates, allowing monthly wages for the provision of victuals; the inmates, supervised by a warden, only dined together on appointed days.

The new model of almshouse, while providing the same standards of privacy and comfort, more or less did away with any kind of accommodation for staff and in time the communal rooms were also to vanish. Compare, for example, the buildings at Audley End with common hall and chapel with that of the hospital founded by William Goddard at Bray in 1627 (**50**). William Goddard provided rooms 'fit and convenient for forty poor

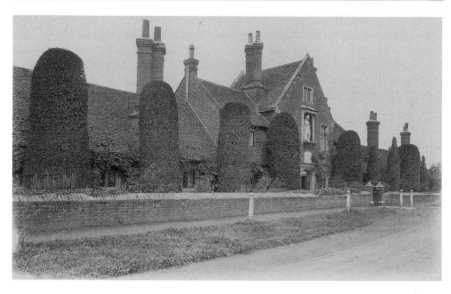

50 Jesus Hospital, Bray, founded in 1627 by William Goddard, a merchant; the more modest version of the courtyard plan with individual dwellings but no communal facilities.

with an apartment each and one kitchen and a bakehouse common to all the poor people' (*PP 1825* 10: 114-18). The absence of a common hall is most marked, and there was no provision for staff accommodation although the hospital is grouped around a courtyard. The Jesus Hospital at Bray is illustrative of the new model of almshouse which arose alongside the more traditional courtyard-plan foundations.

These new establishments most typically consisted of a row or group of dwellings distinguished by the absence of any form of collegiate or monastic type facility. Inevitably there could still be found establishments which were a mixture of the old and the new. Few foundations were built with accommodation for staff, but on occasion a row of dwellings retained a chapel, such being included in the building of Ingram's Almshouse in York, founded in 1632 by Sir Arthur Ingram (**51**). Although these York almshouses suffered damage in the Civil War and have since been modernized at the rear and in the interior, they present one of the best examples of their kind still to be seen. The building consists of a long row of eleven brick bays of two low storeys with a central four-storeyed tower – in the north-east face of this tower is a late-twelfth-century archway from the priory of the Holy Trinity. The single-storeyed chapel projects back from the tower.

Another very fine foundation, with central chapel, is the almshouse at Wimborne St Giles, the gift of Sir Anthony Ashley and built in 1624 (**52**). The building comprises a substantial single-storeyed red-brick range of

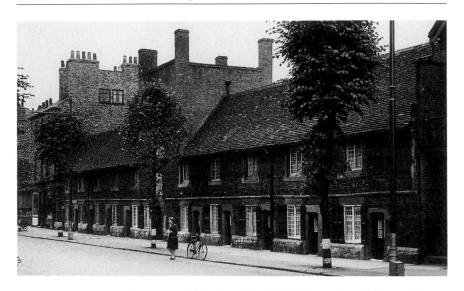

51   Sir Arthur Ingram's Hospital, Bootham, York (1624), a substantial row of dwellings retaining an integral chapel.

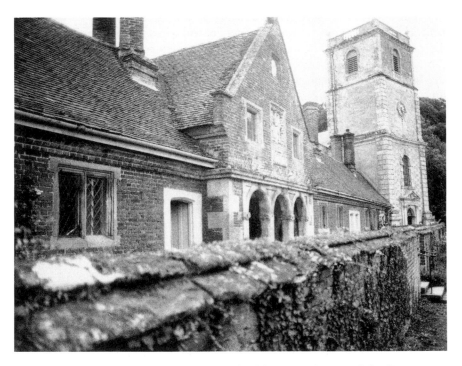

52   The Ashley Almshouses at Wimborne St Giles, a single row of dwellings frequently to be found, as here, adjoining the parish church.

ten dwellings, five on either side of the chapel. There was originally a room over the chapel, probably used as a common room but demolished in 1958 when the original altar was removed to the church porch.

However, it had become unusual for this type of almshouse to possess a chapel. After the Reformation, the religious services prescribed for use in a chapel ceased, and even at several of the older foundations such as the hospitals of St John the Baptist, Winchester, and Bablake's at Coventry, the chapel fell into disuse. It was never to regain its pre-eminence. Where provision for prayers was made, it was more likely to be in an ordinary room specially set aside for the purpose as, for example, at the Trinity Hospital, Aylesford (1600), or in a room that the warden might 'think fit' as at the Hext almshouses at Somerton (1626).

As the chapels disappeared, so too did the resident priests and their houses. In some of the old foundations like St Bartholomew's, Sandwich, no regular provision was made for a priest after the Reformation, and by 1630 one of the brothers was directed to say prayers every morning, bury the dead and church the women, with a minister being provided three or four times a year to administer the sacraments. Likewise in the new foundations, as at Aylesford, one of the inmates was usually expected to be able to read prayers morning and evening. An inmate of the Maison Dieu at Melton Mowbray (*c.* 1640) was paid 10s. per annum for reading prayers in the almshouse on Wednesdays and Fridays. This may have been common practice since literacy, particularly the knowledge of the Lord's Prayer and Creed, was frequently cited as a condition of entry in the almshouses of the late sixteenth and early seventeenth centuries.

More often the inmates were directed to attend the local parish church. The statutes of Lathom Hospital, Oundle (1620), ordered the inmates

> every Saboth and weeke day com to the church yf the Bell doe ring or tole to prayer, on payne to forfeit for every defaulte one peny (Melville 1899: 32).

At Sir Edmund Wright's foundation at Nantwich (1638), the inmates were to attend the parish church twice daily and pray for the flourishing estate of the Commonwealth, bless God for their founder and pray for his posterity. In comparison with the attendance at divine offices expected of the inmates of Ewelme in the fifteenth century, attendance at church was much reduced, ranging from Sundays, Wednesdays, Fridays, Saturdays and holidays at Farnham, to a mere Sunday at the Jesus Hospital, Rothwell (1591). The inmates of Sir John Kidderminster's almshouses at Langley Marsh had a particularly close connection with the parish church since not only were they directed to attend its services but they were also responsible for keeping clean the chapel within the church and its vault.

The almshouses at Langley Marsh adjoin the south side of the churchyard. It is a special feature of these smaller almshouses, built without chapels, that they are situated close to the parish church or even adjoining it, as at Donyatt (1624), Poltimore (1631) and Wimborne St Giles (1624). Indeed, to accommodate the many disabled or enfeebled almsfolk, it was essential for the church to be within easy walking distance – hence the many picturesque groupings of church and almshouse.

The parochial settings of these almshouses were echoed in the provincial character of their foundations. The flood of foundations following the Act of 1597 were often due to the generosity of local men, and foundation charters frequently cited local residence as a qualification for admission. It is this type of foundation that was most usually of the simplest design. A typical example is the Deane almshouse at Basingstoke, consisting of a simple row of eight tenements, with no hall or chapel, under one roof with a central gable. It was founded *c.* 1607 by Sir James Deane, a member of the local gentry, for eight inmates, six from Basingstoke and two from the parish of Dean and Ashe. The almshouses were also administered locally, being placed under the superintendence of the bailiffs, churchwardens

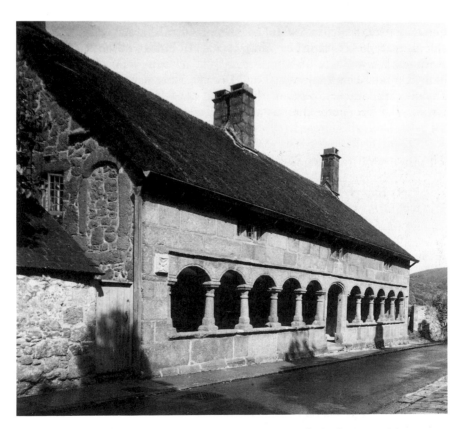

53 The simple row of almshouses at Moretonhampstead, the basic provision commonly found from the seventeenth century.

and the parson of Basingstoke. Other charmingly simple yet differing examples may still be seen at Moretonhampstead founded *c.* 1637, a two-storeyed building separated from the road by a low wall supporting a row of columns (**53**), at Hereford in the one-storeyed timber-framed building of the Aubrey almshouses founded in 1630 (**54**) and at Ross-on-Wye where Rudhall's almshouses, founded in 1575, constructed of red sandstone with gabled dormers lie close to the church (**55**).

Many other small almshouses of the late sixteenth and early seventeenth centuries consist of a similar simple row of dwellings. Occasionally more elaborate designs can be found. One of these was William Cawley's foundation at Chichester (1625), planned in the form of an E with an attractive stepped central chapel (**56**). Another was the Countess of Derby's foundation at Harefield (*c.* 1636), which took the form of an H. The foundations at Chichester and Harefield, although they had no hall, were built on a more ambitious scale. But more often these simple foundations were humble and unpretentious and could be erected easily and relatively cheaply in response to the chronic problem of poverty.

Nevertheless the fact that so many survive today is a tribute to the quality of their building. One of a series of attractive buildings of Cotswold stone, also to be found at Chipping Camden (**37**), Mapledurham, Newbold, Northleach and Winchcombe, remains at Marshfield (**57**) where Elias Crispe, a skinner who became an alderman of London, purchased land in 1625 in his native town on which he erected eight substantial stone cottages for the 'perpetual harbouring of eight poor householders of the

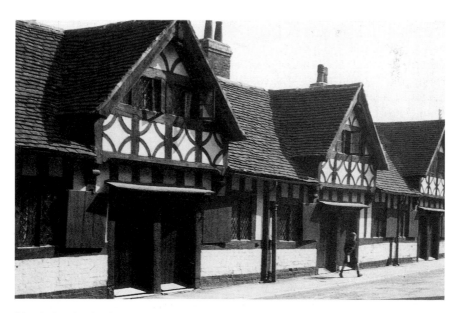

54   Aubrey's almshouses, Ross-on-Wye (1630)

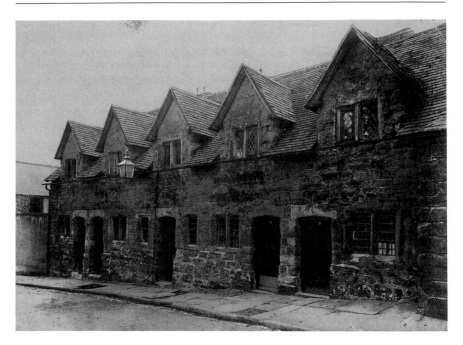

55 Rudhall's Almshouses, Ross-on-Wye, dating to 1575 and early version of the simple row of dwellings.

town and parish' (Jordan 1960b: 149). Many of these smaller foundations were the gift of merchants or tradesmen, especially those who, having succeeded elsewhere, turned to the foundation of an almshouse in their native parish for the perpetuation of their name, while also fulfilling a preceived social obligation. Another fine example from the Cotswolds survives at Wotton-under-Edge (**44**). The original range facing the street has six gables, each with a finial, and a central domed cupola. It was founded by Hugh Perry, a mercer, born in Wotton-under-Edge but Sheriff of London in 1632. He bequeathed £300 for the mayor and burgesses of Wotton to erect an almshouse for six poor men and six poor women. This charitable deed was commemorated in an inscription over the doorway:

> Founder Hugh Perri, squire and alderman of the city of London, borne in this town and besides this gift gave many other good gifts for the good of this town. AD 1638 (*PP 1826-27* 10: 347-52).

Inscriptions were a common way, in these foundations, of ensuring the remembrance of the founder. They might vary from the mere placing of the initials (for example, TD on the shields in the spandrels of Thomas Dutton's almshouses at Northleach) to the simple inscription over the gateway at Ilton: 'This house was founded by John Wetstone, gentleman,

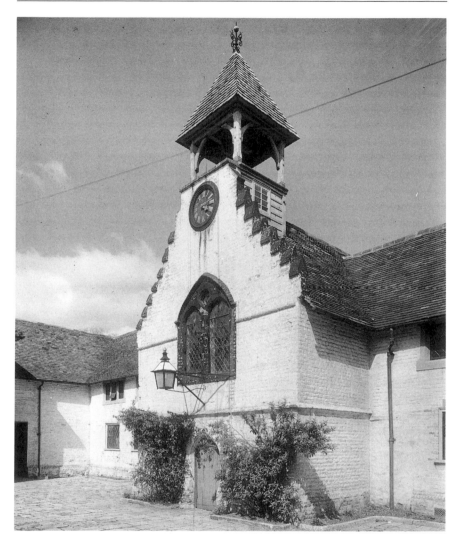

56 Cawley's Hospital, Chichester (1625), planned as an E shape with central chapel.

for the relief of the poor of Ilton in 1634', or to the greater elaboration of the Sedley's almshouse at Aylesford: 'This house was founded by the right worshipful Sir William Sedley, knight, heir and sole executor unto his brother John Sedley, esquire for the relief of ten poor persons with the like allowance, for ever, six at the charge of John Sedley and the residue of the said Sir William Sedley. Finished *primo Aprilis Anno Dni*, 1607.'

The Sedleys further embellished their almshouse of Holy Trinity at Aylesford by placing the family arms over the centre door (**58**). This form of decoration, also to be seen at Sir Stephen Soame's foundation at Little

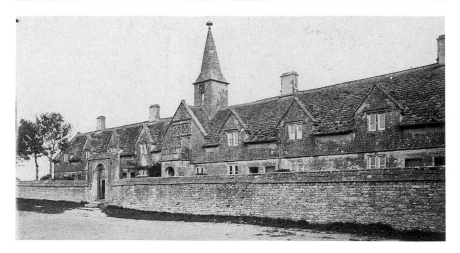

57   The almshouses at Marshfield, one of a number of similar seventeenth-century establishments still to be found in the Cotswolds.

Thurlow, was another popular and relatively inexpensive way of commemorating the founder and his family and frequently the gild company of which the founder was a member. The simple row of almshouses at Baldock, founded in 1621 by John Wynne, citizen and mercer of London, is decorated by an inscribed panel with the shields and arms of the founder and of the Mercers' Company. Few, however, went as far as John Greenway, founder of the Greenway almshouses at Tiverton (1529), where the chapel is covered with a mass of sculpture depicting the personal devices of the founder (**59**). Greenway was perhaps emulated by John Waldron whose almshouses also at Tiverton (1579) are similarly adorned. At the Long Alley almshouses, Abingdon, refounded in 1580, the portraits of many of the masters survive in the hall. This practice began, according to the former master, Little, writing in 1625, 'that their memories may yet remain lively and continue, the masters and Governors have caused their pictures to be made (or at least so many of them as they could get the portraiture of), and have placed them in the Hospital hall, in fair large tables, and long lasting colours which precedents posterity shall do well to imitate and follow' (Little 1627: 95). Yet another example comes from the almshouses at Farncombe (1622) where the founder, Richard Wyatt, carpenter of London, chose to be recalled for posterity not only by the common practice of the placing of an inscription and coat of arms but also by the commissioning of a remarkable set of effigies of himself, his wife and their six children.

At Farncombe, Wyatt's effigies were placed in the chapel as there was no hall — few of these small foundations contained a hall in the traditional manner. Even in some of the larger foundations, the use of the hall was

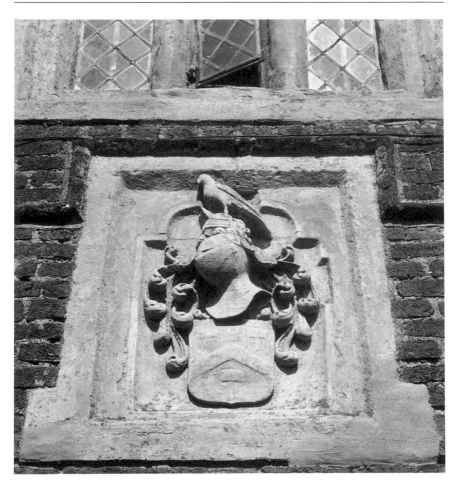

58 Decoration with coats-of-arms was a popular form of personal commemoration as seen over the Holy Trinity Hospital, Aylesford, founded by William Sedley in 1607.

restricted as at the Trinity Hospital, Clun, where the hall and kitchen were reserved for the private use of the warden except on certain named feast days. When a hall was retained for use in the simpler foundations, its lack of status was reflected in the term most often applied to it: an ordinary 'room', specially set aside, as featured in the Duke's almshouses at Bottesford (1612) and, as early as 1580, in the Bedford almshouses at Watford.

Where foundations were equipped with a hall, it was still likely to be the only room with a fire. An interesting example can be found at the Frieston Hospital, Kirksthorpe, founded 1595. The building is of a most unusual design, consisting of a rectangular dining hall surrounded on three sides by the dwellings of the inmates. The doors of the dwellings open into the

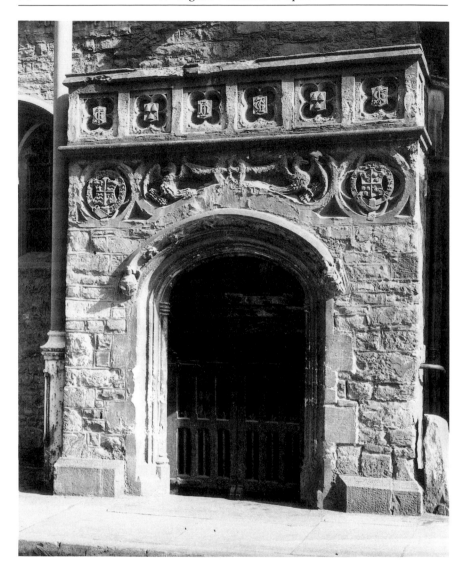

59 The mass of sculpture on the chapel of John Greenway's almshouse in Tiverton depicating the personal devices of the founder.

hall which had a fireplace at one end. There was also clearly only one fire in the hall of Lathom's Hospital, Oundle, for the regulations were quite firm in providing that each inmate should warm in turns at the fire which was kindled at the 'descressione of the Warden' (Melville 1899: 33).

But elsewhere the provision of private chambers, where both sleeping and dining took place, complete with large brick or stone individual chimney-stacks, rendered the hall largely obsolete. Surviving chimneys at

Scutt's almshouses at Cheriton Fitzpaine (1594), John Kidderminster's foundation at Langley Marsh (1617), and the old almshouses at Stoneleigh (1594), to name but a few, show that by the seventeenth century the provision of individual chimneys had become almost a standard feature. Several founders, like Thomas Webbe of Ross-on-Wye (1612), stipulated by will that each of his almspersons was to have not only a separate chamber but a chimney in every chamber. Katherine Wrott, of Sutton-at-Hone, instructed her executors so to construct the building that each of the four almspeople to be maintained would have one chamber above the other and a chimney.

With the increased provision of chimneys, more inmates were encouraged to prepare their own meals either at their fireside or in a common kitchen, and to dine at their own hearth. The decline in the importance of the hall is well illustrated by what occurred at St Nicholas Hospital, Salisbury. Around 1610, the common hall, situated at the east end of the building, was turned into a common kitchen. By this date the brethren at Salisbury were probably self-providing, and few inmates of the newer simpler almshouse foundations were provided with total maintenance or were fortunate even to dine at the house of the founder, as they did at Sir Roger Manwood's hospital in Canterbury (1570). Many were paid an annual sum, for example £3 per annum at Christ's Hospital, Firby, £8 per annum at Perry's almshouses, Wotton-under-Edge, to provide for their own victuals and other needs.

The garden

With the growing emphasis on self-provision, the importance of the almshouse garden increased markedly. Of course, there had always been gardens and orchards producing food for the community. But from the fifteenth century the significance of the garden increased as it became the responsibility of individuals. As early as 1395/6, John Barnstaple, founder of the Holy Trinity Hospital, Bristol, allotted twelve gardens to the twelve inmates of his hospital, a practice much in evidence in the post-Reformation foundations. It is also clear that the permanent inmates at the Newarke, Leicester, had been given a garden that they certainly valued, for in 1440 they complained that it was worth 8s. a year to them but one of the prebendaries had broken down the fence and was using it as a stable. The inmates of God's House, Ewelme, were fined if they failed to clean up the courtyard and weed their gardens.

In the post-Reformation hospitals the special requirement of a garden was made quite clear. Katherine Wrott, of Sutton-at-Hone, as well as providing each inmate with a chimney, also instructed her executors that each inmate should share in a common garden. And there are many other similar stipulations included in the founding statutes of almshouses elsewhere. One of the most detailed examples comes from the Pemberton almshouses at St Albans, where the will of the founder recited that he had purchased a close to build an almshouse for six poor widows with 'six sufficient rooms and six convenient garden plots to be walled with brick or stone and each garden to be divided from the other by sufficient pale' (*PP 1833* 18: 207). At Broadway, the founder, Alexander Every, ordered his 'convenient' gardens to be of a particular length – 12.2 m as they remain today (Jordan 1960a: 54).

The most interesting example and clearest indication of the rising importance of the garden is revealed at the Long Alley almshouses, Abingdon. In 1625 the master gives a succinct account of the improvements carried out to the garden in 1590:

> . . . the Masters and Governors, since the foundation of the hospital (1580) have enclosed and annexed a garden plot to the said almshouses on the west side thereof, where before was nothing but stinking ditches and filthy dunghills, very unwholesome and noisome to the poor people. This plot they have cleansed, manured, dressed and made it fruitful ground, and new ditched it about and caused fair sweet water to run by it, they fenced it with a quick mound and planted the borders with fruit trees and allotted each of the almsfolk a portion of the ground to bear them herbs for their use and flowers for their pleasure, and so, the place that was offensive and noisome before is now become healthy and profitable for them (Little 1627: 93-5).

Gardens also provided another important amenity, especially for the smaller complex – that of an alternative to the hall, in poor weather, for exercise. An early example comes from the almshouse at Walthamstow (1515). Here a close of 0.8 ha was purchased adjoining the almshouses, specifically set aside for the inmates to grow their crops, dry their clothing and 'take their recreation' (Jordan 1960a: 140).

Walthamstow also provides an example of a feature most often associated with the later foundations – the incorporation within the foundation of a free school. At Walthamstow a space was set aside in the upper storey of the almshouse for a schoolroom and an apartment for the schoolmaster. An earlier example of this social obligation can be found at William de la Pole's foundation at Ewelme where the buildings of the school adjoin the hospital to the west. After the Reformation it was quite common for a school to be attached to a hospital, for example at Oundle (1569), St Thomas the Martyr, Canterbury (1620), and Whitgift's foundation at Croydon (1596-7).

CHAPTER SIX

LEGACY AND EVOLUTION

This study of the standing remains of medieval hospitals and almshouses has shown a great change in their nature and design from *c.* 1100 to *c.* 1640. The plans, always of practical design, served to fit a particular requirement. As circumstances and demands changed, so too did the hospital, adapting to meet differing conditions and needs.

The earliest hospitals, founded in the twelfth and early thirteenth centuries, had to provide a building suited to the task of furnishing a temporary refuge for the poor, sick or the traveller and, at the same time, ensuring a spiritual haven for the short-term and longer-term inmates. The needs of the inmates were met by staff following a monastic rule. One of the primary tasks of both the inmates and staff was to pray for the soul of their founder. These considerations determined the design of the earliest hospitals.

As excavations at Ospringe have shown, these early hospitals shared many similarities in their layout with the contemporary monastic complex, providing spiritual and domestic accommodation for both staff and inmates. But, very definitely, the focus of the early hospital foundations was the infirmary hall and chapel. Plans of the foundations of this date and surviving buildings, like St Mary's at Chichester, show that, as with the monastic infirmary, the plan was governed by the need to accommodate both the temporal and the spiritual requirements. Indeed the spiritual needs were paramount. The design had to allow easy access to an altar for those sick and unable to leave their beds. This resulted, for many of the larger foundations, in a standard plan of a communal infirmary hall, sometimes aisled and with adjoining chapel. These hospitals were admirably suited to their task and the success of the arrangement can be measured in its continuance at many of the more old-fashioned establishments throughout the later Middle Ages.

Responding to the special importance attached to the spiritual side of these foundations, architectural emphasis in the early hospitals lay in their chapels. The chapels were subject to frequent attention and alteration and were rarely allowed to fall into ruin. Many fine examples of hospital chapels are still standing, like the elaborate chapel of St Cross near Winchester, or the simpler but still impressive twelfth-century chapel of St Mary Magdalen, Stourbridge, Cambridgeshire. These survivals bear witness to high quality and to the pre-eminence of ecclesiastical over domestic architecture, an emphasis which continued up to the Dissolution and which is shown particularly well in the sumptuous design and fittings of the late chantry chapel of St Mark's Hospital, Bristol.

Nevertheless, from the late twelfth century there were already changes in the domestic architecture of many of the early foundations. Although the basic plan was retained, the traditional open infirmary-hall arrangement was altered. As early as the mid-thirteenth century some infirmary-hall foundations included private rooms. As would become common practice at late medieval monastic houses, the hospitals were also beginning to divide their infirmary halls into private cubicles. Already in the fourteenth century, the small thirteenth-century foundation of St Mary Magdalen had the aisle space of its infirmary hall partitioned. Further changes were made in the fifteenth century when these cubicles were converted into individual dwellings.

The multiplication of private apartments in the infirmary-hall type of hospital was common from the late twelfth century. Private rooms with the provision of considerable hospitality, as received by Sir Philip Wem at Ospringe, almost certainly had always existed in the medieval hospital, either for longer-term corrodians or for the more favoured members of the staff. The structural changes which took place at Glastonbury and elsewhere, undoubtedly reflected changes in the nature of the foundation. Hospitals increasingly took on the character of almshouses, serving the needs of the longer-term inmate in place of the short-term poor inmate or traveller. The new permanent inmates, who often paid for the privilege, clearly required a higher standard of living than the inmate needing a temporary refuge. The hospitals changed accordingly. The detailed inventory from St Mary's Hospital, Dover, in 1535, listed a variety of private apartments and their furnishings. In addition, the fine quality of the finds from such apartments, excavated at Ospringe and dating from the thirteenth century, shows that hospitals, no less than monasteries, had become accustomed to the higher standards of comfort and privacy also to be found in contemporary domestic architecture.

Nowhere can this be better seen than in the masters' houses. Fine examples of improved lodgings and accommodation, as at Ledbury, were in plain contravention of the spirit of the rule. Like their monastic counterparts, the masters' houses were distinguished by separation from the building housing the inmates. Rooms were partitioned and fireplaces and garderobes installed, emphasizing the increase in standards of comfort and the growing importance of privacy.

Such improved domestic standards are most easily seen in the hospitals and almshouses which were founded after *c.* 1350. The larger hospitals, like the monasteries, succumbed to the economic problems of the fourteenth century and many fell into decline or ruin, or suffered years of mismanagement. From this date the hospitals, with the exception of the Savoy, had mostly become places of refuge for permanent inmates, almsfolk or bedes-men. Any new buildings had to reflect this need. At the same time, late-thirteenth-century and fourteenth-century donors increasingly favoured the smaller institutions of the friary and parish church, or responded to changing conditions by the foundation of smaller, easier to control hospitals or almshouses, better suited to fewer, long-term inmates.

These inmates were likely to demand, for the new foundations, the improved standards of living seen elsewhere. Nevertheless, it was the infirmary-hall type of plan, favoured for its practical design and still suitable for its purpose, that continued to be chosen by a number of founders for their establishments. Founders still instructed inmates to pray for their souls and this required easy and frequent access to the chapel. The new buildings fulfilled these demands. Exemplified by the foundations at Sherborne and Higham Ferrers, these buildings were smaller, more compact versions of the traditional infirmary hall, consisting of a small narrow hall retaining an adjoining chapel. However, as was the case with all foundations after *c.* 1350, the hall was divided upon first building, whether by cubicles as at Stamford or wooden partitions as at Higham Ferrers. Thus greater privacy was assured while retaining the emphasis on the spiritual function of the foundation by continued access to the chapel.

Without doubt, the right to privacy had become customary and had increasingly usurped the ideals of the common life. Private apartments threatened the old-style communal hall. The spiritual life was also eroded by the emergence of a new style of establishment founded after *c.* 1350. Alongside the new, smaller infirmary-hall type of foundation, arose a new type of almshouse which reflected the improvement in individual standards of living seen throughout the later Middle Ages; this was also to be seen in the towns with their provision of paving, drainage and common latrines, and in domestic architecture by the multiplication of rooms which were heated by side-wall or end-wall fireplaces and the provision of garderobes.

These developments are to be seen most clearly at major new-style hospitals like St Cross Hospital, Winchester. St Cross emulated new collegiate establishments and the plans already seen at contemporary manor-houses, with the new buildings erected around a courtyard. These buildings demonstrate the high domestic standard which an inmate of a later medieval hospital had come to expect. Significantly the dwellings were now totally separate, with individual access sheltered by a covered way or cloister. Even more important for ease and comfort, each group of dwellings was provided with chimneys and garderobes. Great chimneys of stone or brick, like those still to be seen at St Cross and outside the hospital of St John the Baptist, Lichfield, were a marked characteristic of this type of foundation and further hastened the demise of the common hall.

The quadrangular plan selected for St Cross, with the accent on comfort and privacy, was also chosen for William de la Pole's foundation at

Ewelme. In contrast to the early infirmary-hall type of foundation, the emphasis in the new hospitals was upon providing a higher standard of domestic accommodation for the inmates. The masters still had superior lodgings, but there were few resident staff and only rarely is there found evidence of the large complex of buildings, like the monastic precinct, that characterized the earlier foundations. Both Ewelme and St Cross retained a hall and chapel, but far less importance was attached to the architecture of the chapel. Indeed, at Ewelme the hospital was attached to an already parish church and the inmates used an aisle of the church. In both foundations the chapel was separate from the dwellings. The inclusion of a chapel ensured that the spiritual nature of the foundation retained its importance. However, by making a distinction in its buildings, separating the spiritual from the temporal and increasing the emphasis on the secular nature of the foundation, many of these hospitals escaped dissolution.

After the Dissolution, with the forced decline of the spiritual function of the hospitals, increased secularization of the buildings had to take place. It is significant that at foundations like Ewelme and St Cross, where there had always been less emphasis on the spiritual side of the buildings, fewer changes were made. Greater changes had to be made in the surviving infirmary-hall type of foundation; of the traditional type, a number like St Nicholas, Salisbury, and St Giles, Norwich, underwent considerable modifications. At Norwich, secularization was achieved by inserting floors in both chapels and turning them into chambers. At the same time standards of comfort and privacy, long familiar in some of the hospitals, were improved by inserting an extra floor into the infirmary hall and by the provision of chimneys. Elsewhere, the old-style infirmary-hall design was considered inadequate and, as at God's House, Southampton, new standards, which promised considerable comfort, were introduced by the provision of an entirely new set of buildings adjacent to the old.

The changes and new standards introduced at the later medieval hospitals were continued in the foundations which sprang up after *c.* 1560. The courtyard plan, familiar from the pre-Dissolution foundations, continued to be favoured. These foundations provided similar high standards of privacy and comfort. Although chapels were still provided in some foundations, like the Trinity Hospital at Croydon, they were of little significance, with less emphasis upon attendance and frequently no resident priest.

Very little emphasis was now placed on chapel architecture and with individual dwellings a standard feature, the hospitals and almshouses founded after *c.* 1560 afforded ideal vehicles for personal display. As Cardinal Beaufort had done at St Cross in the fifteenth century, so John Whitgift, Archbishop of Canterbury, at the Trinity Hospital, Croydon, furnished his foundation with a massive gatehouse. Both gatehouses survive as lasting memorials to their founders. Certainly, one of the characteristics of the post-Dissolution foundation is this emphasis on display by the founder. No longer could the chief duty of the inmates be to remember their founder in prayer. But his memory was ensured by a proliferation of personal embellishment in the form of coats of arms, shields, initials and effigies, none more conspicuous than those of Sir Thomas Coningsby at Hereford.

Even the smaller foundations, dating from the second quarter of the seventeenth century, usually included at least an inscription on their walls. These hospitals or almshouses were cheaper to build and easier to control, but continued to ensure remembrance of their founders, usually men of lesser means, often merchants or tradesmen. They arose alongside the larger courtyard-plan foundations and were a marked contrast to anything which had gone before, reflecting a response to changed expectations and fulfilling an urgent need. Simple in design and plan, they most typically consisted of a row of terraced dwellings, characterized by an almost complete lack of any form of communal building.

Despite their simplicity, all were equipped to the same high standards of the larger courtyard-plan foundations. All were provided with private chambers and often chimneys, as did Katherine Wrott for her foundation at Sutton-at-Hone, prescribed by will or deed. Gardens were also common, encouraging self-provision and helping render the common hall obsolete.

Just as the bedesfolk no longer gathered together to eat communally, so they were unable to attend their own private chapel. Rarely was a chapel provided in these small foundations, although inmates were normally expected to attend the local parish church which was often adjoining or within a short walking distance. Any pretence of a communal life had disappeared. The new almshouses, consisting of simple single-rowed dwellings, catering for the long-term secular inmate and still much in evidence today, were a mere shadow of the great infirmary halls of the early Middle Ages with their communal halls and elaborate chapels.

GAZETTEER

AVON

Bristol: Forster's almshouses

Forster's almshouses and their chapel dedicated to the Three Kings of Cologne, were founded in the early 1480s by John Forster. The almshouses were intended for a priest and thirteen almspeople. In 1577 the foundation was conveyed to Thomas Colston, mayor of Bristol, and other members of the corporation. The foundation was well supported by the burgher aristocracy of Bristol during the sixteenth and seventeenth centuries.

The almshouses originally comprised fourteen rooms each with a garden plot but now only the fine Perpendicular chapel which adjoined them remains.

Bristol: St Bartholomew's

St Bartholomew's Hospital was founded in the thirteenth century by John de la Warre for the maintenance of two chaplains, brethren and sisters. By 1340 the hospital was ruled by a prioress with sisters. In 1412 an inquisition decided that the hospital ought to be ruled by men who were secular priests. In 1445 the character of the foundation changed again when a fraternity of twelve poor mariners was established there with a priest. But in 1531 Lord de la Warre conveyed the hospital and all its property to Robert Thorn to enable him to found a free grammar school.

There remain only a few thirteenth-century fragments of the hospital including an archway, two trefoil-headed arches and a defaced statue of the seated Virgin.

Bristol: St Mark's

St Mark's or Gaunt's Hospital was founded *c.* 1220 by Maurice de Gaunt as an almonry attached to St Augustine's Abbey, for the feeding of 100 poor people every day and the maintenance of a chaplain to pray for the souls of Maurice and his ancestors. The foundation was administered by the abbey until 1232 when Gaunt's nephew, Robert de Gurnay, made it an independent foundation. Numbers declined in the later fourteenth century, and there were accusations in 1406 and 1438 that the feeding of the poor had again been neglected. A series of disputes concerning the patronage of the house, quarrels with its powerful neighbour, the abbey of St Augustine, and conflicting claims on the endowment raged throughout its history. The endowment was always slender and it was dissolved in 1539.

The chapel of St Mark dates from the thirteenth century with many additions and alterations. The impressive Poyntz chapel was completed in 1536.

BERKSHIRE

Abingdon: St Helen's or Christ's Hospital

The almshouses at Abingdon, originally dedicated to St Helen, were founded in 1446 by the influential and wealthy Fraternity of the Holy Cross. They were intended for thirteen 'impotent' men and women and two priests. The fraternity was closely connected with the church and no inmate was to be admitted without the consent of its members.

The foundation flourished alongside the fraternity until the latter was dissolved in 1547. Nevertheless, the Crown continued to support the almsfolk until the foundation was created a corporate body by royal charter in 1553. It was thenceforward to be known as Christ's Hospital and was endowed with the remaining possessions of the old fraternity supplemented by properties that had formerly belonged to the abbey of Abingdon. The master and twelve governors, chosen from the better inhabitants of the town, were entrusted with the administration of the establishment, the functions of which had been increased to provide relief to the poor inhabitants of the town and to the local grammar school, as well as perpetual sustentation of seven men and six women.

The almshouses form an attractive row of tenements with central hall, running along the western edge of St Helen's churchyard. They were built in 1446 as thirteen separate dwellings, although little of that date remains visible on the outside. The chief feature of the exterior is the wooden cloister, probably added *c.* 1500, running along the whole eastern façade with three porches added in 1605. The porches were decorated with 'satyrs and antiques', which have since disappeared. The octagonal lantern was also added about this time but restored in the eighteenth century. Much of the interior was also remodelled in the early seventeenth century. The stone mullioned bay window of the hall was constructed in 1605 **(60)** and oak panelling added in 1606-7; the Jacobean oak table was made for the governors in 1608. The gardens to the rear were enclosed and laid out in 1580.

Abingdon: St John the Baptist

The hospital of St John the Baptist is said to have been built by Abbot Vincent of Abingdon Abbey (1117-30). It probably remained under the

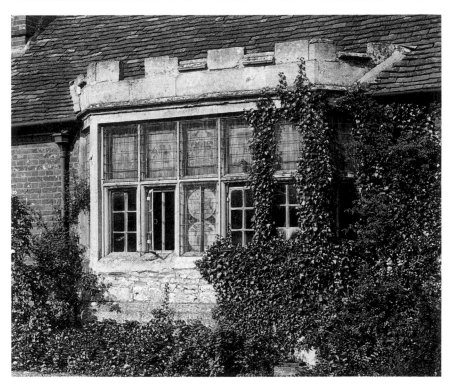

60 The bay window of the hall of St Helen's Hospital, Abingdon, reconstructed in 1605.

patronage of the abbey since the master or prior of the hospital was appointed by the abbot. The foundation prospered during the thirteenth century but was dissolved with the abbey in 1538. The buildings were sold to the town corporation in 1561.

The hospital was situated at the gate of the abbey, and the guildhall which now adjoins the abbey gatehouse incorporates part of the hospital chapel, the only surviving building. The chapel was sited in the north range of the hospital. The other buildings were demolished and reused for the erection of the free grammar school in 1652.

Bray: Jesus Hospital

Jesus Hospital was founded by William Goddard, a wealthy London fishmonger and native of Bray. His foundation was for forty poor. The buildings were completed in 1628.

The buildings comprise forty low cottages of brick in the form of a large quadrangle. Each cottage has one room and between every two rooms is a common vestibule entered from the courtyard. At the back, each cottage has a separate doorway. The centre of the eastern range is two-storeyed with the chaplain's lodgings over the entrance. Opposite, in the centre of the western range, stands the chapel. A statue of the founder stands in a niche above the entrance and on either side are the arms of the Fishmongers' Company and Goddard.

Donnington: God's House

The God's House Hospital at Donnington was founded or refounded in 1393 by Sir Richard Abberbury, guardian of Richard II. In 1503 the hospital was forfeited to the Crown, the latter appointing the masters until 1514 when the Donnington estates were granted to Charles Brandon, Duke of Suffolk. In 1547 the hospital was again taken by the Crown and remained Crown property until 1600 when it was granted to Charles Howard, Earl of Nottingham. Howard refounded the institution in 1602 and it was hence known as the hospital of Queen Elizabeth.

The hospital was situated 0.8 km from the parish church adjoining the castle. The almshouses were probably completely rebuilt by Charles Howard between 1600 and 1602. They consist of a series of one-storeyed, red-brick individual dwellings with a covered way around a small courtyard. A larger room called the hall was set aside for common use.

Lyford: The almshouses

The almshouses at Lyford were founded in 1611 by Oliver Ashcombe, for ten poor persons and a minister who was to read prayers and have a room in the house.

The buildings, much modernized, are constructed of brick and form a quadrangle with the chapel situated on the west side.

Newbury: St Bartholomew's

The foundation date of St Bartholomew's hospital is unknown, but it first appears in the records in 1215 when King John granted it an annual fair. From the early fourteenth century, the prior was appointed by the towns-people; the last prior is recorded in 1547 after which the town took over the management of the hospital.

In the second half of the sixteenth century there was said to be a chapel with a door leading to a house on the south side, and over the body of the church were two chambers with chimneys. But the house was pulled down and four small tenements were built to maintain four almsmen. The chapel was converted into a schoolhouse and the remains consist of a plain rectangular room with gabled roof in which there are elaborately carved and moulded queen post trusses.

Thatcham: Loundre's almshouses

The Loundre almshouses were founded before 1446 by Thomas Loundre for poor travellers and lame soldiers returning homewards.

To the north of the chapel stands a three-storeyed, three-bayed house of brick, possibly that of Loundre's foundation.

BUCKINGHAMSHIRE

Buckingham: St John the Baptist
The hospital of St John the Baptist was founded in the late twelfth century by William Frechet for the poor and infirm. Soon after its foundation it had ceased to fulfil its original purpose and in the mid thirteenth century it was sold to the Archdeacon of Buckingham who resumed its use as a hospital. In 1279 it was granted to the foundation of St Thomas of Acon, London, whence it became a chapel and chantry.

The chapel of St John the Baptist and St Thomas of Acon still stands close to the parish church. It retains a Norman south doorway but the remainder was entirely rebuilt *c.* 1475.

High Wycombe: St John the Baptist
Little is known of the history of the hospital of St John the Baptist but it was probably founded *c.* 1180 and may have belonged, originally, to the Knights Templars and then to the Knights Hospitallers. By 1344, the patronage was in the hands of the mayor and burgesses. In 1548, there was a master, but no brethren, maintaining three beds for poor and infirm travellers. At the time of the suppression of the chantries, the hospital was sold to the corporation and the buildings converted for use as a grammar school.

Within the school grounds are the ruins of some of the hospital buildings. Part of an arcade built *c.* 1180 remains and probably formed part of the hall, estimated to have been 19 m long and 5 m wide. To the south-east of this arcade is a wall of later date which may have been the chapel.

Hughenden: The almshouses
The almshouses at Hughenden were probably founded in the early seventeenth century by Sir Robert Dormer (died 1616). The Dormer family had been in possession of the manor of Hughenden since 1540.

The almshouses stand to the south-west of the church and consist of a row of four cottages. They were extensively remodelled in 1842 and only one original timber-framed gable remains on the front; there is more timber-framing to the rear. The interior has exposed beams and a large open fireplace.

Langley Marsh: The almshouses
The almshouses at Langley Marsh were founded *c.* 1617 by Sir John Kidderminster and were intended for the support of two poor men and two poor women of the parish.

The almshouses stand south of the church and consist of a rectangular block, built of brick, and divided into four tenements. On the north side the upper storey is situated in the four gables and has mullion head and diamond patterned windows. There is another gable over a central porch of two storeys, faced with cement. The entrance arch has a tablet over it with the arms of Kidderminster and inscribed with the date 1617. A central chimney-stack of brick, set diagonally, and two similar stacks, project at each end of the building.

Wing: Dormer's Hospital

Dormer's Hospital at Wing was founded in 1596, as stated on a tablet in front of the building, by 'Dame Dorothy Pelham sometime wife to Sir William Dormer, Knight, Lord of the manor of Wing'. It was intended for eight poor persons.

The almshouses, situated 274 m south-east of the church, are built of stone rubble and brick and consist of one storey with an attic. There are gables at each end and dormer windows in front and to the rear of the four tenements. Each tenement was intended to be occupied by two persons. The almshouses were much remodelled in the nineteenth century.

CAMBRIDGESHIRE

Ely: St John Baptist and St Mary Magdalen

A hospital in Ely is referred to in the Pipe Roll for 1169 but it is uncertain to which institution this refers. The hospital of St Mary Magdalen first appears in the records in 1225. The hospital of St John Baptist was probably also in existence at this time, for the two hospitals were united by Bishop Northwold in 1254. By the mid fifteenth century the hospital had fallen into poverty and ruin, and by 1500 seems to have become a sinecure free chapel. The hospital escaped dissolution until 1561 when it was granted to Clare College.

Documentary evidence reveals that, in the fourteenth century, the hospital consisted, at least, of chapel, infirmary, refectory, dormitory and cloister. Now there are only the remains of two chapels. The chapel of St Mary, converted to a dwelling after 1561, probably continued in use after the hospitals were united. It is the largest of the remaining buildings and more ornate. There are signs of the existence of a north and, perhaps also, a south aisle, and there may have been a chancel. The chapel of St John, a smaller plainer building, was possibly converted to use as a barn shortly after the amalgamation of the hospitals.

Huntingdon: St John the Baptist

The hospital of St John the Baptist was founded by David, Earl of Huntingdon, probably in the mid thirteenth century. Little is known of the history of this hospital, but after the Reformation the foundation continued as a school with part of its endowment used for the maintenance of almshouses for the relief of travellers and sick persons.

The two western bays of the nave of the hall survive, now incorporated within a museum.

Peterborough: St Thomas the Martyr

The hospital of St Thomas the Martyr was founded at the gates of the monastery by Abbot William of Wateville, and completed and endowed by Abbot Benedict (1177-94). The foundation was intended for the support of bedeswomen and eight were being maintained there in 1535. The hospital was treated, from the first, as part of the possessions of the abbey almoner and was dissolved with the abbey in 1539.

The chancel of the hospital still exists, dating to *c.* 1330. The chapel was also used by the parishioners of Peterborough. The chapel, situated on an embankment, was reached by a series of steps. On either side of the entrance, built into its structure, was a shop and there were seven other shops between the corner of the building and the gate of the abbey.

Ramsey: St Thomas the Martyr

The hospital of St Thomas the Martyr was probably founded *c.* 1180 although little is known of its history. By the fourteenth century it had become a parish church.

In the course of its history as a parish church, various additions and alterations have been made to the basic twelfth-century hospital which consisted of a small chancel with north and south chapels and a nave of eight bays with north and south aisles.

Stourbridge, By Barnwell (Cambridgeshire): St Mary Magdalen

The hospital of St Mary Magdalen was probably founded in the first half of the twelfth century but it does not appear in the records until 1169. It was intended for the reception of lepers. By 1279 it was no longer carrying out any eleemosynary function and probably continued in existence as a free chapel until the fourteenth century when it ceased to be used for worship.

The chapel survived as a storage place for the local fair. It has been carefully restored and now provides one of the most complete examples of Norman hospital architecture.

Whittlesford Bridge: St John the Baptist

The hospital of St John the Baptist was founded before 1236 possibly by Sir William Colville who gave the patronage to the Bishop of Ely. Little is known of its history, and by 1337 it was a sinecure free chapel.

The chapel is the only remaining building and is a fine example of thirteenth-century hospital architecture, consisting of chancel and nave without structural division.

CHESHIRE

Nantwich: Wilbraham's almshouses

The Wilbraham almshouses were founded by Sir Roger Wilbraham some time in the sixteenth century. Little else is known of their history.

The almshouses form a sixteenth-century timber-framed range of two low storeys.

Nantwich: Wright's almshouses

The Wright almshouses were founded by Sir Edmund Wright, Lord Mayor of London, but native of Nantwich, shortly before 1638. His foundation was intended for the relief of six poor men, to be aged fifty years or more and conforming to the religion of the Church of England.

The almshouses consist of six substantially built brick cottages of two storeys with mullioned windows. An archway to the front garden has two large volutes and Tuscan columns were added in 1666. The whole building was dismantled and re-erected on a new site in 1975.

CORNWALL

Lanivet: St Benet

The history of the hospital of St Benet at Lanivet is obscure but it was probably founded in 1411 as a leper house. By the sixteenth century, the hospital had been converted into a manor-house belonging to the Courtenay family.

The mansion with its façade of 1859 contains some earlier features belonging to the hospital and, situated to the rear of the house, is most of the tower of the original chapel.

St Germans: The almshouses

The almshouses at St Germans were founded in 1583 by Sir Walter Moyle, then the head of the principal family in the parish.

The almshouses, built with roughly squared blocks of granite, form an attractive composition, originally consisting of twelve dwellings, six on the ground floor and six above. Five gables project on to the street front and are supported on tall stone piers, thus permitting a gallery to each floor. The upper floor is reached by an open stairway.

Truro: Almshouses

The almshouses at Truro were founded by Henry Williams, a linen draper of the town, and others, described as gentlemen, for the habitation, sustentation and relief of ten poor people.

The buildings, with inscription, still stand but are much altered.

DERBYSHIRE

Ashbourne: The Field almshouses

The Field almshouses were founded by Roger Owfield, a London fish-monger, who died in 1607 leaving £100 for the building of an almshouse for eight poor people of the town. The foundation was completed by his widow in 1630 for a further £76.

The almshouses, situated close to the church, comprise a row of eight two-storeyed tenements under one roof. They are constructed of stone and have four-centred doorways, low mullioned windows and plain gables.

Etwall: Etwall Hospital
The Etwall Hospital was founded in 1590 by will of Sir John Port whose family held the manor. He directed his executors to provide an almshouse to be built near the church for six poor.

The two-storeyed buildings form three sides of a courtyard. The doors and windows on the ground floor of each house are stone-framed but plain brickwork is exposed in the gables.

Wirksworth: Gell's bedehouses
Gell's almshouses at Wirksworth were founded by Anthony Gell in 1579. The foundation was intended for six poor men of Wirksworth.

The almshouses, situated near the school and fronting the churchyard, stand very much as they were built in 1584. They consist of six dwellings, three on the ground floor and three above with three-light mullioned windows and gable ends. A brass inscription placed on the outside of the almshouse reads as follows: 'This almshouse was founded onlye at the costes and charges of Anthony Gell late of Hospton Esq. deceased in the year of our lord God 1584 and twentie pounds by year give for ever by the said Anthony Gell for the relieffe of sixe pore impotent men in the same almshouse. Yf thou wilt O!Lord please helpe y pore in ther disease.'

DEVON

Cheriton Fitzpaine: The almshouses
The almshouses in Cheriton Fitzpaine were founded in 1594 by Andrew Scutt for six poor of the parish.

The buildings are of cob construction with thatched roofs and prominent stone chimneys.

Exeter: God's House
God's House or Wynard's was built by William Wynard, recorder of Exeter, in 1436 for twelve poor, infirm and elderly men. Wynard resided in his almshouses until his death. The foundation escaped dissolution and the mayor of Exeter was appointed visitor.

The almshouse dwellings were destroyed during the Civil War and the buildings now on the site mostly date from 1836. However, the original chapel survives; built along the street front, its most noteworthy architectural feature is the elaborately carved arch separating the nave from the chancel.

Exeter: St Katharine's

The hospital of St Katharine at Exeter was founded in 1457 by will of John Stevens, canon residentiary of St Peter's cathedral, for thirteen poor persons.

Of the hospital buildings only the outer walls of the chapel remain.

Moretonhampstead: Almshouses

The almshouses at Moretonhampstead were probably founded *c.* 1637, but little is known of their history.

The almshouses comprise a two-storeyed building constructed of large, squared granite blocks with a thatched roof. On the ground floor, the rooms open on to a narrow terrace which is separated from the road by a low wall supporting a row of columns. The windows are mullioned, those on the upper storey set under the projecting eaves.

Poltimore: The almshouses

The almshouses at Poltimore were founded by John Bamfylde, in memory of his wife and son, in 1631 for the poor of the parish of Poltimore.

The almshouses adjoin the churchyard and consist of four two-storeyed dwellings under one roof with a central gable. The buildings are much restored.

Taddiport (Little Torrington): St Mary Magdalen

The hospital of St Mary Magdalen may have been founded by Ann, daughter of Sir Thomas Esteler, Earl of Ormond, for lepers. Very little is known of its history, but it was not dissolved and by 1665 had become an almshouse.

The hospital chapel, dating from the mid fourteenth century, remains. It consists of a small nave and north-east transept with a small tower at the west end.

Tiverton: Greenway's almshouses

The Greenway almshouses were founded in 1529 by John Greenway, a wealthy merchant of Tiverton. His foundation was intended for five poor men unable to work for a living, and not having the wherewithal to provide themselves with food, drink and clothing.

The almshouses comprise a single row of three storeys with three rooms in each, but they were much altered in the nineteenth century. The chapel adjoins, its most distinctive feature being the porch with its mass of sculpture.

Tiverton: Waldron's almshouses

The Waldron almshouses were probably founded by John Waldron, a wealthy merchant of Tiverton.

An inscription over the gateway of the almshouses bears the date 1579 and the whole edifice is covered with the personal devices of John Waldron. The building, comprising eight small rooms, has a wooden gallery along the front with the entrances at the rear. Under the gallery runs the inscription: 'Depart thy goods whyl thou hast tyme, After thy deathe, they are not thyne. God save Queen Elizabeth.' Adjoining is the chapel with a porch containing many sculpted motifs in Perpendicular style.

Tiverton: Slee almshouses

The Slee almshouses at Tiverton were founded in 1610 by George Slee for the maintenance of six poor single women, inhabitants of the town, to be aged over sixty years.

A low range of almshouses with wooden gallery remains, although much restored.

DORSET

Bridport (Dorset): St John the Baptist

The exact date of foundation of the hospital of St John the Baptist at Bridport is unknown, but it was in existence by the early thirteenth century when there were a warden or prior, brethren and sisters. Very little is known of its history but it seems to have been under the patronage of the bailiffs and commonalty of Bridport who, in 1357, granted it to John de Shapwick, chaplain, on condition that he maintained daily services in the chapel. The foundation was dissolved in 1547.

The only surviving building is a humble stone structure of the sixteenth century with one oriel window.

Dorchester: Napper's Mite almshouses

Napper's Mite almshouses were founded in 1615 by Sir Robert Napier, the son of a Dorset family and Member of Parliament for Dorchester in 1568. The foundation was intended for the habitation and maintenance of ten poor men.

The almshouses are now a shopping centre but the original foundation comprised ten apartments and a chapel in the form of a small quadrangle. The front block has a cloistered walkway with a staircase leading to a large room on the second floor, possibly the former common hall.

Pamphill: St Margaret and St Anthony

Little is known of the history of the hospital of St Margaret and St Anthony at Pamphill, but it probably began as a leper house in the twelfth or thirteenth century. By the sixteenth century, the building had been converted to almshouses.

The single-storeyed row of almshouses are constructed of cob with thatched roof and date no earlier than the sixteenth century. Next to the almshouses is the original chapel of the hospital; a simple structure of nave and chancel in one.

Poole: St George's almshouses
The St George almshouses were probably erected by the Gild of St George, a religious fraternity; they were founded at the end of the four-teenth century for the poor members of the gild. The almshouses first appear in the records in 1429, but little is known of their history. They were granted to the corporation of Poole in 1604.

The buildings may date from the early fourteenth century. It is possible that they were originally single-storeyed. A projecting upper storey was added in the early sixteenth century, with the upper rooms approached from the street by a long flight of steps. This upper storey was cut away in 1904 when the building was much restored. The sixteenth-century timber roof is still well preserved inside.

Sherborne: St John the Baptist and St John the Evangelist
The hospital of St John the Baptist and St John the Evangelist was originally founded in 1406 but refounded by licence of Henry VI in 1437. The foundation was intended for the support of twenty brethren, twelve poor men, four poor women and a chaplain.

The buildings were completed in 1448 and form a particularly well-preserved example of a two-storeyed infirmary hall with chapel at the east end. The chapel contains some contemporary stained glass and an exceptionally fine late-fifteenth-century triptych. The chapel continues through both floors, communicating with the infirmary hall through a screen on the ground floor and a stone arch on the upper. The position of small windows in the wings either side of the hall, westwards of the entrance, suggests that these may have been the original situation of the brethren's apartments with a dining hall at the west end. Externally, the south front, with its two storeys of seven one-light windows and octagonal chimney-stacks, presents a fine façade.

Wimborne: St Margaret and St Anthony
The hospital of St Margaret and St Anthony was founded in the early thirteenth century for lepers. Little is known of its history and it was dissolved in 1547 but refounded from 1567.

The hospital is situated about 0.4 km to the north-west of the town. The buildings consist of a chapel, dating from the early thirteenth century, adjoined on the east by the much modernized tenements of the almspeople.

Wimborne St Giles: Ashley almshouses
The almshouses at Wimborne St Giles were founded in 1624 by Sir Anthony Ashley in gratitude for recovering from a serious illness. Over the entrance is a quotation from Psalm 54: 'He hath delivered me out of all trouble.' The foundation was intended for eleven poor and needy persons.

The almshouses are attached to the north-west corner of a church of a later date. They comprise a single-storeyed red-brick range of ten one-roomed dwellings, five either side of a recessed, gabled central bay which contained the chapel and a room over. A sculpted coat of arms of the Shaftesbury family decorates the gable under which is a three-bayed stone arcade of classical type. The almshouses are raised above the village green and are separated from it by a terrace and low brick wall.

DURHAM

Durham: St Giles
St Giles Hospital was founded by Bishop Flambard of Durham in 1112 for the poor. The original building was burned down during a feud over the bishopric in 1144. After 1153, the hospital was rebuilt on a new site by Bishop Pudsey and given a fresh constitution for a master and thirteen brethren who were to live under monastic vows. Difficulties were experienced in the fourteenth century: in 1306, the Scots set fire to the hospital and burnt down the muniment room and there were charges of maladministration in 1311 and 1347. The hospital also suffered from the Black Death through death of tenants, lack of thraves and tithes, and loss of 600 sheep. By the mid fifteenth century, the revenues had so fallen that it was not possible for the hospital to maintain the buildings and continue to provide hospitality. By 1532 there was another charge of wastage of goods and misappropriation of funds and in 1535 the staff was reduced to four chaplains and two lay clerks and only ten permanent inmates were supported. The hospital surrendered in 1545.

Only St Giles church survives from the original hospital; the north side of the nave, an impressive piece of Norman architecture, dates to Bishop Flambard's foundation. A fine gatehouse with vaulted gateway with rooms above it and to the sides, built by Bishop Bury in 1341, survives from the rebuilt foundation. There is documentary evidence of an extensive twelfth-century complex including a church, hall, infirmary, dormitory and a court but nothing of this now remains.

Durham: St Mary Magdalen
The hospital of St Mary Magdalen was possibly founded by Sir John Fitz Alisaundre in the mid thirteenth century for a chaplain and thirteen men and women. Little is known of the history of this hospital except that by 1534 there were only three brethren and two sisters. When Durham Priory was dissolved and the new cathedral established, the hospital lands were leased out.

The ruins of a large rectangular chapel remain. This was the chapel erected anew and consecrated in 1451. At its east end is a fourteenth-century decorated window which must have been transferred from the former chapel.

Friarside

The foundation date of this small hospital is unknown but it was in existence by 1312 when a master was appointed. Little else is known of its history except the names of some of the masters. In 1439 Bishop Neville appropriated it to the chantry of Farnacres.

The hospital was situated on the south bank of the river Derwent but all that remains today is the shell of the fourteenth-century chapel.

Gateshead: St Edmund, the Bishop and Confessor

This hospital was founded in 1248 by Nicholas Farnham, Bishop of Durham. The foundation was for a master and three priests. There is no mention of any poor inmates, and an inventory of 1325 reveals no accommodation for the sick, so the hospital may have existed solely to provide temporary relief for the poor and travellers at its gate. The 1325 inventory indicates a prosperous hospital and by this date it had been united with the older hospital of the Holy Trinity. In 1348 the hospital was given to the nuns of St Bartholomew's, Newcastle, for their support and it remained in their possession until they were both dissolved in 1539.

After the Reformation, a mansion was built on the site of the hospital and only the chapel of the buildings, recorded in 1325, remained. In 1746 the mansion was burned down and in 1837 a new church, dedicated to the Holy Trinity, was erected on the site with the old chapel being restored and incorporated in it as the south aisle. The west front of the chapel stands almost as it was built in 1248 and represents a fine example of Early English architecture.

Sherburn: St Lazarus, St Martha and St Mary Magdalen

The hospital at Sherburn was founded *c.* 1181 by Bishop Pudsey for a master, three priests, four clerks and sixty-five leprous persons. In 1314, the foundation was reconstituted by Bishop Kellaw providing for four priests and four clerics. By 1429 the establishment was destitute and grave complaints were made as to its management. Bishop Langley instituted an inquiry and procured a bull authorizing another reconstitution of the hospital. One of the reasons for its decline was that few leprous persons could be found, so the new statutes, promulgated in 1434, provided for an establishment consisting of four priests and four clerks, as before, but the number of lepers was reduced to two, if they could be found, and thirteen poor men were also to be maintained with an honest woman engaged to care for the sick. However, in 1501, the master expelled the sick and grave abuses occurred in the administration of the hospital revenues during the reigns of Henry VIII and Edward VI. Nevertheless, the foundation was not suppressed and from 1552 many of the evils were remedied. By Act of Parliament in 1585 the establishment was incorporated, to be known as Christ's Hospital for the maintenance of thirty brethren.

Very little of the original structure remains. The south wall of the chapel and part of the tower contain work dating to the foundation of Bishop Pudsey and much of the rest of the chapel may have been rebuilt following the original design. The entrance gateway is also ancient, containing a pointed tunnel vault inside, crossed by heavy transverse ribs.

Witton Gilbert: St Mary Magdalen
The hospital of St Mary Magdalen at Witton Gilbert was founded in the second half of the twelfth century by Gilbert de la Lay, lord of the manor of Witton, for the support of five lepers. Very little is known of its history but it was dissolved either with the priory in 1540 or in 1547 with the chantries and gilds.

A few features of the hospital survive in Witton Hall, including a fine fourteenth-century decorated window, probably part of the chapel.

ESSEX

Audley End: College of St Mark
The college of St Mark was originally founded as an almshouse at the end of the sixteenth century by Thomas Howard, first of the Howard earls of Suffolk. The foundation was for twenty poor men. It was dissolved in 1633 by the Countess of Suffolk who found herself unable to maintain it.

The buildings are of brick, planned around two courtyards, with the centre range containing the common hall and with the chapel at its east end. Surrounding each courtyard are ten dwellings.

Harlow: Stafford almshouses
The Stafford almshouses at Harlow were probably founded in 1630 by Alexander Stafford, but nothing else is known of their original constitution.

The buildings comprise three two-storeyed half-timbered tenements under one roof, standing east of the parish church. The doorway and windows have original shaped brackets with supporting hoods and a similar bracket supports the eaves gutter. The upper storey projects at the rear.

Ilford: St Mary and St Thomas the Martyr
The hospital of St Mary and St Thomas the Martyr was founded *c.* 1140 by Adeliza, sister of the Abbess of Barking, and came under the patronage of that abbey. The foundation was originally intended for the support of thirteen leprous servants or tenants of the abbey. However, by 1397, only one poor man was maintained. In 1535, there were two poor men and a priest. The hospital was not suppressed but was taken over by the Crown. In 1572 Queen Elizabeth granted her rights as patron to Thomas Fanshawe, Remembrancer in the Exchequer.

Of the hospital buildings, only a chapel, drastically restored in the nineteenth century, remains. The chapel was probably rebuilt in the late fourteenth century, but only the chancel is basically of that date.

Maldon: St Giles

The hospital of St Giles was founded some time before 1164, probably by a king of England. An inquisition of 1402 recorded that it had been founded for the maintenance of a chaplain and the leper burgesses of the town, but there had been no lepers there for twenty years. In 1481 Edward IV granted licence for the patrons to grant the hospital and all its possessions to the abbot and convent of Beeleigh. The hospital remained in the possession of Beeleigh Abbey until they were both dissolved in 1536.

The hospital remains are scanty but form what seems to have been quite an ambitious structure. They consist of part of the transepts of a chancel chapel probably dating to the end of the twelfth century. Early-thirteenth-century lancet windows are to be found in the south transept.

Rochford: Rich almshouses

The Rich almshouses at Rochford were founded in 1567 by Richard, Lord Rich, for six poor almsmen.

The buildings consist of a one-storeyed brick range with two gabled accents. They are divided into six one-roomed tenements with small gardens attached.

GLOUCESTERSHIRE

Chipping Camden: The almshouses

The almshouses at Chipping Camden were founded in 1612 by Sir Baptist Hicks, a wool merchant, for twelve persons.

The almshouses consist of a raised terrace of two-storeyed buildings situated close to the parish church. They are symmetrical in plan with gabled bays.

Cirencester: St John the Evangelist

The hospital of St John the Evangelist was probably founded *c.* 1133 by Henry I for the sick and destitute. Throughout its history the hospital was closely associated with the abbey of Cirencester but it was not suppressed.

A Norman arcade of four bays with a cottage built into one of the bays still survives. This originally formed part of an aisled infirmary hall built in the twelfth century. A chapel was added in the fourteenth century.

Cirencester: St Thomas's

St Thomas's Hospital was founded in the mid fifteenth century by Sir Wiliam Nottingham for four decayed weavers.

The two-storeyed medieval stone building has small rectangular windows and a four-centred archway with a defaced image above.

Gloucester: St Bartholomew's

St Bartholomew's Hospital probably began as a hostel for workmen who were building the bridge over the river Avon. When the bridge was finished they remained and gave hospitality to travellers and cared for the sick. It was certainly well established when Henry II gave it a charter and an endowment of lands in 1220. During the thirteenth century the hospital was well supported, but by 1343 the hospital was described as 'much decayed'. There were also several commissions inquiring into maladministration in the second half of the fourteenth century. By 1380, the situation had so deteriorated that the prior and brethren were reported as having taken away the beds of the sick, made a door in the house of the poor through which they drove their pigs and unroofed another great house of the poor. Nevertheless, the hospital continued to survive and was not suppressed at the Reformation, but in the reign of Elizabeth the poor of the hospital petitioned the queen about the parlous state of the foundation. An agreement was made in 1564 between the queen and the mayor and burgesses, amounting to a second royal foundation, whereby the hospital was repaired and new chambers built. The new foundation was intended to support one priest, one physician, one surgeon and forty poor.

Nothing remains of the old buildings of the hospital, but a drawing of 1780 made shortly before demolition shows a fine example of Early English architecture. Archaeologists have also been able to reveal some interesting features of the hospital plan which complement the documentary history. Excavations have shown an infirmary hall of seven bays with the further two bays forming what has been described as the 'nave' of the hospital chapel, with the chancel added slightly later. It is unusual to find a hospital chapel with both nave and chancel attached to an infirmary hall of this type. It is possible that the 'nave' was the original chapel attached to an infirmary hall of seven bays, which, as the hospital prospered and increased in size during the thirteenth century, was enlarged and a new chapel added.

Marshfield: Crispe almshouses

The Crispe almshouses were founded by Elias Crispe, alderman of London, on land purchased in 1625 in his native town. They were intended for eight poor householders of the parish.

The almshouses, built of Cotswold stone and standing at the entrance to the town, form a striking structure of eight two-storeyed cottages under one roof, four either side of a gabled chapel. Over the chapel is a double panel enclosed by a framework of classical columns with base and entablature; above this rests an unusual miniature square tower and spire. The almshouses retain their original two-light mullioned windows and have four chimney-stacks and small walled gardens. They are separated from the road by a brick wall with a tall entrance gateway.

Newland: The almshouses

The almshouses at Newland were founded in 1617 by William Jones, a haberdasher of London and staunch Puritan, for the habitation of eight poor men and eight poor women of the parish. Governance was entrusted to the Haberdashers' Company.

The almshouses are situated along the south side of the churchyard. They consist of a low range of ten two-storeyed tenements (some were double apartments). There were originally ten doors on the ground floor, but some have been converted to windows, with small windows on the upper floor. There are also five sets of grouped chimneys.

Northleach: Dutton almshouses

The Dutton almshouses were founded in 1616 by Thomas Dutton, who devised lands to his brother to erect six two-storeyed houses, each with a separate garden.

The almshouses, built of Cotswold stone, form an attractive two-storeyed symmetrical building with steeply pitched gables and mullioned windows. Each doorway gives access to two houses and the centre one bears the initials of Thomas Dutton on the shields of the spandrels. Each house contained a brass plate inscribed with the letter D.

Winchcombe: Chandos almshouses

The Chandos almshouses at Winchcombe were built by Lady Dorothy Chandos.

The almshouses are situated to the south of the church. Built of Cotswold stone, they comprise a plain two-storeyed range of twelve tenements, six on each floor. The arms of Chandos of Sudeley are displayed on the façade and the entrances are situated at the rear of the building.

Wotton-under-Edge: Hugh Perry's almshouses

The almshouses at Wotton-under-Edge were founded in 1630 by Hugh Perry, a native of the town and leading member of the Mercers and East India Company, for six poor men and six poor women, to be aged at least fifty years.

The almshouses, built in 1638, form an attractive two-storeyed building of Cotswold stone originally arranged around three sides of a courtyard with six gables on the street façade. An inscription on the front reads: 'Founder Hugh Perri, squire and alderman of the city of London, born in this town and beside this gift gave many other good gifts for the good of this town. AD. 1638.' A central passageway in the front range leads to the small courtyard which is almost filled by the chapel.

HAMPSHIRE

Fordingbridge: St John the Baptist

The origins of the hospital of St John the Baptist at Fordingbridge are obscure but it was in existence by 1272, possible having been founded by one of the lords of the manor of Nether Burgate, but by that date was under the control of the bishops of Winchester. The foundation was granted by Cardinal Beaufort to his new establishment at St Cross Hospital in Winchester but although the property of St Cross was not confiscated at the Dissolution, by 1570 the hospital of St John the Baptist was in private hands.

There only remain the fragmentary ruins of the hospital standing close to the river Avon on the south side of the town.

Odiham: Almshouses

The almshouses at Odiham were founded in 1623 by Sir Edward More of Odiham. They were intended for the habitation of eight poor persons.

The almshouses were built on a site immediately south of the church. They form a picturesque group of one-storeyed houses of red brick, forming three sides around a small courtyard. The entrance façade has a gabled wing and an archway in the centre with a passage through to the courtyard; the rooms lead off this passage. Substantial chimney-stacks project from the exterior of the tenements.

Portsmouth: God's House

God's House Hospital, Portsmouth, also known as the hospital of St John the Baptist and St Nicholas, was in existence just before 1214 when it was granted a charter by King John. The house was intended to accommodate travellers, sick and aged people. It was under the management of Southwick Priory until 1316 when the advowson was granted to the Bishop of Winchester. From 1305 the masters were absentees or pluralists, and in 1539 there were said to be only six poor men maintained in the hospital. The foundation was dissolved in 1540.

Of the original hospital buildings, only the church remains. It consists of an aisleless nave (now roofless) and chancel separated from the nave by a screen. The chancel probably dates from the time of the foundation *c.* 1212-20 and the nave slightly later. The building was thoroughly restored in 1886.

Southampton: God's House

God's House Hospital, also known as St Julian's, was founded *c.* 1197 by Gervase and intended for the poor and travellers. In 1238, the wardenship was taken by Queen Eleanor and conferred upon Crown nominees. From 1293 until the hospital was granted to Queen's Hall, Oxford in 1343, the wardens were absentees. Nevertheless, the establishment was never in debt and seemed to be well administered. The hospital was burned by the French in 1338 and was rebuilt at least once after this date before being replaced by almshouses in 1588-93. The new almshouses were intended for four brethren and four sisters. A steward was appointed to administer the establishment and its estates and he lived in a house which was rebuilt in 1588-93, incorporating part of the domestic buildings of the old hospital that were no longer required.

Up to the mid sixteenth century, the foundation had possessed all the buildings necessary to maintain the inmates of a normal religious house with halls, chapel, chambers and domestic buildings. The hall was later incorporated into the steward's house but it is not clear how many of the other buildings survived the 1588-93 reconstruction. The almshouses consisted of two, two-storeyed rectangular blocks. The chapel survived the 1861 demolition and was restored but it is still basically that which was built with the hospital *c.* 1190, consisting of nave and chancel with original chancel arch. The tower was the entrance to the hospital with a blocked fifteenth-century doorway. Major work was carried out on the chapel between 1423 and 1424.

Winchester: Christ's Hospital
Christ's Hospital at Winchester was founded in 1607 by Peter Symonds, a mercer, for the support of six poor men, one poor woman and four homeless boys.

The hospital is set back from the road, separated from it by a narrow garden. The red brick buildings, comprising a central block of three storeys linked by two long wings, are divided into small tenements. In the central block is a small stone tablet with a sculpted coat of arms and an inscription. 'Peter Symonds, Founder, 1607'.

Winchester: St Cross
The hospital of St Cross at Winchester was founded in the mid-twelfth century by Bishop Henry de Blois, possibly on the site of an older foundation. It was intended for the relief of 13 poor men and for the provision of daily doles to 100 men of good conduct. Henry de Blois granted control of the hospital to the Knights Hospitallers, but after his death a series of disputes over the government of the institution continued until 1303 when control finally rested in the hands of the bishopric. The struggle for power was followed by a series of serious abuses in administration of the hospital by the masters, and by the time Bishop William of Wykeham took a close interest in the affairs of St Cross in 1372, the 100 poor had been removed to a hovel at the gate and the 13 inmates ejected from the buildings. Under the influence of Wykeham and the work of his nominees Nicholas of Wykeham and John de Campedene, the spiritual life of the hospital was restored and its buildings repaired and improved.

Wykeham's successor to the bishopric was Cardinal Henry Beaufort, half-brother of the king and four times lord chancellor. Beaufort only began to take an interest in St Cross during the last years of his life (died 1447), when he decided upon a scheme of expansion, adding to the original foundation a new institution distinct from de Blois' hospital but under the same master. The new foundation was intended to provide for two priests, thirty-five brethren and three sisters, men or women of gentle birth who had lost their wealth or former members of Beaufort's household. It became known as the hospital or almshouses of 'Noble Poverty'. In 1461 when the Yorkist party gained permanent power Yorkist claimants to the St Cross endowments succeeded in depriving the foundation of its most valuable properties. After 1485 Bishop Waynflete was unable to regain these endowments, and consequently the hospital was refounded in 1486 for only one chaplain and two brethren; it thence seems to have merged with the old hospital and ceased to have an independent existence.

The hospital survived the Reformation but in 1557 there was another scandal when the master disposed of much of the hospital's property. The new master fought a series of expensive legal campaigns to recover the property and succeeded in having an Act of Parliament passed in the reign of Elizabeth to regain the possessions.

The outstanding feature of the buildings of St Cross is the church. It is cruciform in plan and vaulted throughout. There appear to have been four major phases of construction. John de Campedene, master 1382-1410, did much fine work in the church, rebuilding the tower, reroofing the chancel and aisle, installing a considerable amount of glazing and paving, enclosing the Lady Chapel for the brethren and inserting a high altar of alabaster and a painted reredos. He was buried in the church and a magnificent monumental brass perpetuates his memory. The woodwork in the choir dates to the thirteenth century.

Marks on the south and east walls of the church and a blocked-up doorway in the south transept seem to indicate that the domestic buildings of the original hospital lay to the south of the church, but no trace of them remain above ground. However, the Hundred Men's Hall may be the building now standing on the east side of the outer, smaller quadrangle.

The buildings of the inner quadrangle, as they now stand, were erected in conjunction with the foundation of Cardinal Beaufort *c.* 1445. The quadrangle is entered by a massive three-storeyed gatehouse. The west range and former south range (demolished 1789), contain the brethren's lodgings. The east range, with ambulatory, was remodelled at the beginning of the sixteenth century and a second storey added in the seventeenth century.

Winchester: St John the Baptist

The hospital of St John the Baptist at Winchester was in existence by 1270. The hospital was under the control of the corporation for much of its existence and although the foundation was taken into Crown hands at the Dissolution, it was not suppressed and was regranted to the corporation with only the chapel having fallen into disuse. In 1558, Ralph Lamb bequeathed £400 to the master and brethren to maintain as many poor as the bequest would support. Six poor and needy widows were admitted to six almshouses erected in a court on the north side of the main buildings. The foundation was granted a new charter by Elizabeth in 1588.

The chapel and porch of the hospital remain. Excavation has also revealed the plan of the ground floor of the main building which was divided into two by a spinal wall. The southern part adjoined the chapel and was probably the infirmary hall, while the northern part may have been the domestic side. The entire structure was of one build, probably dating, as do the porch and chapel, to the fifteenth century and most likely represents the rebuilding and reroofing ordered by the town corporation in 1408.

HEREFORDSHIRE

Hereford: Aubrey's almshouses
The Aubrey almshouses were founded and endowed by the will of Mrs Mary Price in 1630 for six poor women.

The almshouses consist of a block of six one-storeyed tenements with attics. The building is timber-framed with three symmetrically placed gables on the street front with moulded bressumer and barge-boards. The doorways, in pairs, are also moulded. Three chimney-stacks project from the rear.

Hereford: Coningsby Hospital
The Coningsby Hospital exists on the site of the hospital of St John which was founded some time after 1221 and had become the property of the Knights Hospitallers *c.* 1340. This hospital was dissolved in 1540 and was refounded in 1614 by Thomas Coningsby, soldier, 'in gratitude for protection in his travels by land and sea as well as against malice at home'. The foundation was intended for the support of eleven poor, old soldiers or mariners who were known as Coningsby's Company of Old Servitors, one old soldier was the master, known as the Corporal.

The buildings are arranged in a quadrangle incorporating the thirteenth- and fourteenth-century remains of St John's Hospital. These remains are now only seen in the north range which contains the hall and chapel. The hall and chapel were partly reconstructed in 1614 when the other three ranges, consisting of twelve two-storeyed dwellings for the inmates, were added together with the original great gateway which stood at the south end of the street front and formerly led to Sir Thomas Coningsby's house but now separate from the quadrangle. The Corporal was to have the lodging adjoining the hall and the chaplain the lodging adjoining the chapel. Carved in the walls of the chapel are various heraldic devices of the Coningsbys and a stained-glass window depicts the family's arms. The arms are also displayed on a sculpted tablet over the door between the chapel and hall.

Hereford: Lingen's almshouses
The Lingen almshouses were founded in 1609 by Mrs Jane Shelley.

The buildings consist of a half-timbered, single-storeyed range of six tenements, each with two rooms. The front is symmetrical with square-headed doorways in pairs, with a dormer above each pair. There are projecting chimney-stacks to the rear. The almshouses were restored and partially rebuilt in 1801 and 1849.

Hereford: St Giles
St Giles Hospital was founded after 1150, possible originally as an asylum for lepers, but later for the relief of the poor. Very little is known of its history but it was not suppressed at the Reformation.

The present hospital building dates mainly from the eighteenth century, but its foundations date back to the twelfth century. These foundations indicate a rare circular chapel with an apsidal chancel to the east of it. It is possible that the hospital was administered by the Knights Hospitallers whose foundations are characterized by this type of architecture. In the west wall of the hospital there is a reset Norman tympanum.

Ledbury: St Katherine's
St Katherine's Hospital was founded in 1232 by Bishop Hugh Foliot. The foundation was intended for the support of the poor and needy and was to be staffed by brethren and sisters living a quasi-monastic life. However, supervision was often lax and in 1398 a stricter set of ordinances were issued. Nevertheless, the hospital survived dissolution but, in 1580 was granted to Bishop John Scory. The dean and chapter protested and appealed to the court of chancery which restored the hospital to them.

Of the hospital buildings, a barn, master's house and infirmary hall with chapel survive. The infirmary hall dates from *c.* 1330 when a papal indulgence of that date described the hospital as 'new'. Built in local sandstone, the chapel occupied 6.7 m at the east end of the infirmary hall and is separated from the hall by a timber truss. Inside there is an early-seventeenth-century communion table, some stained glass depicting the arms of Bishop Grandisson and various tiles dating to the late fourteenth or early fifteenth century, including representations of the shield of arms of Edward the Confessor and the Beauchamps. The hall is now divided into three rooms with the three eastern bays forming a vestibule to the chapel. At some time a floor was inserted, possibly at the same time as the building of the master's house.

The master's house, constructed partly of timber-frame and partly of brick, was originally built in the fifteenth century and is of two storeys. It has absorbed many alterations and affords examples of domestic architecture of several centuries. It was extended after the valuation of the foundation in the late sixteenth century and altered again in the seventeenth and eighteenth centuries. The accounts of the first master to be appointed, from 1584 to 1595, after issue of the new statutes, show the hospital to be alive with continual building activity with the constant employment of carpenters, glaziers, plumbers, joiners, masons, pargetters, smiths, tilers and thatchers. The original fifteenth-century roof of the hall remains. The former solar wing is lined with late-sixteenth-century panelling with a frieze; the fireplace is flanked by Ionic pilasters and the overmantle has a late-sixteenth-century painting of Bishop Foliot and on the frieze above is the date 1588.

The barn, to the south-west of the hospital, is timber-framed, and was built in the seventeenth century but has been partly reconstructed.

Ross-on-Wye: Pye's almshouses
Pye's almshouses at Ross-on-Wye were founded in 1615 by the Reverend William Pye, Vicar of Foyle. The establishment was not endowed but entrusted to the rector, churchwardens and overseers of the poor.

The almshouses, situated 393 m north of the church, consist of a two-storeyed range of four tenements, originally of two rooms each. They have been much restored.

Ross-on-Wye: Rudhall's almshouses
Rudhall's almshouses were founded in 1575 by William Rudhall for the poor persons of the parish of Ross-on-Wye.

The buildings, situated 55 m north-east of the church, consist of a range of five tenements of two storeys, constructed of red sandstone. The upper windows lie in gabled dormers.

Ross-on-Wye: Webb's almshouses
Webb's almshouses were founded in 1612 by Thomas Webb for seven poor people. Each inmate was to have a separate chamber and a chimney in every chamber.

The almshouses, situated 119 m south-east of the church, comprise seven two-storeyed tenements with walls of stone and timber-framing.

HERTFORDSHIRE

Aldbury: The almshouses
The almshouses of Aldbury probably date from the sixteenth church, but little is known of their foundation or subsequent history.

The buildings adjoin the churchyard and in the nineteenth century consisted of eight small tenements. Before recent improvements, the almshouses formed three timber-framed two-storeyed cottages with thatched roofs.

St Albans: Pemberton almshouses
The Pemberton almshouses were founded in 1624 by Roger Pemberton

for six poor widows who were to be aged at least sixty years and to have had an honest and good life and to have been resident in certain named parishes.

The almshouses stand north of St Peter's church and comprise a single, one-storeyed row, built in red brick and divided into six tenements. They are set back from the road with a garden in front, bounded by a low wall, entered through a tall central gateway over which is an inscription recording that they were founded by Roger Pemberton.

Stanstead Abbots: Baeshe almshouses

The Baeshe almshouses were founded in 1635 by Sir Edward Baeshe for six poor women of the parish.

The almshouses are situated at the entrance to the village of Stanstead Abbots. They comprise a substantial two-storeyed brick building of six cottages under one long, steep roof. The upper windows are set in three gables and the original oak doorposts and moulded oak window frames remain.

Watford: Bedford almshouses

The Bedford almshouses at Watford were founded in 1580 by Francis, second Earl of Bedford, for the habitation of eight poor people from the parishes of Langley and Chenies.

The almshouses comprise two storeys of timber and plaster with five gables on the front. They retain their original window frames and four chimney-stacks of two shafts each. The building consists of sixteen apartments on the ground floor, two for each inmate, with a large common room on the upper floor. A garden behind was divided into eight portions.

KENT

Aylesford: Trinity Hospital

The Trinity Hospital was founded by John Sedley, a member of a prominent local family and considerable benefactor to the charities of Kent. By his will of 1605, Sedley required his executor to build and endow an almshouse for six poor persons. His brother, heir and sole executor, Sir William Sedley, stated by a deed of 1617 that he had carried out his brother's instructions by building a house of stone and had increased the endowment to provide for ten poor men.

The almshouses consist of a gabled row of one-storey cottages, built of Kentish rag, under one roof and with half-dormers in the gables. One room was formerly used as a chapel. Tall chimneys project from the rear of the building which is mostly below ground level. Over the centre door are the arms of the Sedleys and the following inscription: 'This howse was founded by the right wo: Sir William Sedley, knight, heire and sole executor unto his brother, John Sedley, esquire, for the relief of ten poor persons, with the like allowances, for ever, six at the charge of the said John Sedley and the residue of the said William Sedley. Finished *primo Aprilis Anno Dni 1607, Anno regni regis nostri Jacobi quinto. Gloria soli Deo.*'

Canterbury: Jesus Hospital

The Jesus Hospital was founded shortly before 1599 by Sir John Boys for the complete maintenance of between twelve and twenty almspersons.

The almshouses stand by the north gate of the city. They form a U-shaped block, constructed of brick, of two storeys with a central gable.

Canterbury: Manwood's Hospital

Manwood's Hospital was founded by Sir Roger Manwood in 1570 for six poor.

The almshouses form a long two-storeyed brick range of six tenements.

Canterbury: St John the Baptist

The hospital of St John the Baptist was founded and endowed by Lanfranc, Archbishop of Canterbury between 1070 and 1089. It was for sixty poor and infirm persons, thirty of each sex. The house was in financial difficulties in the fourteenth century, but it survived dissolution and in 1560 Archbishop Parker made fresh ordinances.

Lanfranc's hospital was situated outside the north gate of the city and built of stone. The surviving remains of the hall indicate a building probably 46 m long. Part of the south nave of a double aisled chapel, placed in the centre of one side of the hall, still exists. A fragment of a staircase of a later date suggests the insertion of an upper storey, and there is also an interesting Tudor gatehouse on the street which may mark the site of the original porter's lodge.

Canterbury: St Mary's or Poor Priests

The hospital of St Mary or Poor Priests was founded *c.* 1220 by Alexander of Gloucester. It was supported by the abbey of St Augustine throughout its history but it was not suppressed. However, in 1562 Archbishop Parker found it in ruin and decay and it was ceded to the Crown in 1575. The Crown granted the foundation to the mayor and corporation whence it was used as a bridewell for paupers and a school.

The hospital buildings consist of a stone-built hall with solar and service wings and chapel. Excavations have revealed a long history of continual rebuilding and alteration.

Canterbury: St Nicholas and St Katherine

The hospital of St Nicholas and St Katherine, also known as Cogan's, was founded shortly before 1203 by William Cockyn, a citizen of Canterbury. However, as an independent institution the foundation was short lived and was united to the hospital of St Thomas in Eastbridge in 1203 and passed into private hands *c.* 1230.

A dwelling was first mentioned on the site *c.* 1200 and the walls of flint and chalk with stone dressing probably date to before 1200, surviving to roof level except in the front wall. It is likely that William Cockyn added the aisled hall to the rear for the hospital. This hall with part of its roof remaining was probably of two bays, but part of it was pulled down and the façade totally altered in the sixteenth century.

Canterbury: St Thomas à Becket
St Thomas's Hospital was probably founded *c.* 1180 by Edward Fitz Odbold for poor pilgrims. It was later dedicated to Thomas à Becket and its importance increased with pilgrimages to his shrine. In the fourteenth century the hospital suffered poverty and abuses, and in 1342 Archbishop Stratford drew up fresh, stricter ordinances for its governance. The foundation survived the Dissolution and in 1557 was still receiving poor, but by 1576 the hospital was certified as ruinous and let out to tenements.

The chapel, lying parallel to the street, still survives. It is of two storeys and was extended to the east in the fourteenth century. At right angles to the chapel stands the hall with an undercroft dating to *c.* 1180. A timber loft was added in the late sixteenth century.

Chatham: St Bartholomew's
The hospital of St Bartholomew is said to have been founded by Gundulf, Bishop of Rochester (1077-1108) for lepers. Little is known of its history until the foundation escaped dissolution. In 1619 James I granted it to James, Viscount Doncaster, but after a long fight by the patron, the Dean of Rochester, it continued to function as a hospital.

The hospital stood outside the east gate of the town but the chapel is all that now remains. It consists of nave, chancel and apsidal sanctuary dating to the twelfth century with later additions. Recent excavations have discovered the possibility of a medieval hall running east–west from the south wall of the nave.

Cobham: Cobham College
The Cobham almshouses are on the site of Cobham College, founded in 1362, which was suppressed at the time of the Reformation. The buildings and lands remained in the possession of the Cobham family, and it was the intention of Sir William Brooke, Lord Cobham, to rebuild the college and refound it for the relief of the poor. This was not accomplished before his death in 1596 but his will provided instructions for carrying out his design and for endowing the foundation.

The present buildings, completed in 1598, occupy the site of the fourteenth-century college, being built around two quadrangles close to the south side of the church. Around one quadrangle are the almspersons' dwellings, each consisting of a sitting room on the ground floor with a bedroom over. On the south side of this quadrangle was the common hall, which retains its original roof, with a cellar below. The inmates' gardens lay on the east, west and south sides of the quadrangle and there are also the remains of a gateway to the south over which are the founder's coat of arms and a mutilated inscription. Excavations revealed that the new foundation abandoned the former kitchen and that the east and west ranges were reconstructed 1.8 m narrower, and the north range was rebuilt from scratch and a pentice added to the south range.

Dover: St Mary's

St Mary's or Maison Dieu was founded before 1221 by Hugh de Burgh, Earl of Kent and justiciary of England, for the maintenance of the poor and infirm as well as pilgrims. Soon after foundation the patronage was transferred to Henry III. Despite continued grants of gifts and privileges from the Crown, the hospital fell into poverty in the early fourteenth century. One of its burdens was the imposition by the Crown of several corrodies and also, by ancient custom, the chancellor was entitled to have livery for himself and the clerks of the chancery whenever the chancery was at Dover. By 1511, a visitation showed that only a small fraction of its revenues were devoted to charitable purposes and in 1544 the hospital was confiscated.

The buildings which still stand date from the early fourteenth century and comprise a hall set on an undercroft and a tower. The undercroft is vaulted and the hall is spacious, lit by six great four-light geometric windows on the eastern side. The hall was a southwards extension of the twelfth-century hospital, separated from it by a large stone arcade. Nothing remains of the original hall but three bays of the stone-built chapel attached to it can still be identified.

Harbledown: St Nicholas

St Nicholas Hospital was founded *c.* 1084 by Lanfranc, Archbishop of Canterbury. It was founded for sixty inmates, thirty of each sex. By the end of the fourteenth century, only a few inmates were suffering from leprosy but the hospital continued to support the poor. The foundation was not dissolved.

The hospital lodgings and hall were rebuilt towards the end of the seventeenth century, but the church remains and is of considerable interest, showing evidence of continuous alteration. Lanfranc's church was a single-celled apsidal building without structural separation of apse and nave. Not long after foundation, the apse was replaced by a square-headed chancel, narrower than the nave. In the first half of the twelfth century, a short north aisle was added and, in the late twelfth or early thirteenth century, a tower was built to the west of the north aisle connected to the nave by a pointed arch. The north aisle was extended eastwards in the fourteenth century and to the south of the nave a transeptual chapel was added. The chancel arch was removed when a rood loft was erected in the late fourteenth or early fifteenth century. In the fifteenth century, the west wall of the transeptual chapel was removed and a narrower aisle was built extending westwards, with its original door in the end wall giving a separate entrance to the church.

Milton: St Mary the Virgin
The origin of the hospital of St Mary the Virgin is unknown, but it first appears in the records in 1155. The endowment was greatly increased by Aymer de Valence, Earl of Pembroke, in 1321, when he probably refounded the house for a priest master and two chaplains. An inquiry in 1524 found the master and all brethren dead and the king permitted a chantry to be founded in the church.

The church of St Mary still retains the nave and chancel of the hospital, dating basically to the twelfth century.

Ospringe: St Mary the Blessed Virgin
The hospital of St Mary the Blessed Virgin, also commonly called Maison Dieu, was founded probably soon after 1230 by Henry III. It was intended for a master, three brethren and two secular clerks who were to be hospitable to the poor, particularly lepers and needy pilgrims. Almsfolk were also maintained there and the hospital received several royal corrodians. Despite royal support, including continuous exemptions from taxation, the hospital fell into poverty in the early fourteenth century, and in 1330, the king commissioned a visitation as the hospital was reported to be 'greatly decayed through lack of good rule'. The house apparently recovered in the late fourteenth century but its prosperity declined once more in the fifteenth century, suffering badly from plague in 1487 and never recovering. It was finally granted to the Bishop of Rochester in 1516 for the foundation of the College of St John the Evangelist at Cambridge.

The hospital was situated on the main road from London to Dover. The standing remains consist of two small stone undercrofts of the late thirteenth or early fourteenth century, which stand south of the road either side of a stream. These buildings are similar in plan and were probably built to carry first-floor halls. A fairly comprehensive excavation of the site north of the road has revealed buildings which were part of a well laid out monastic-style precinct.

Sandwich: St Bartholomew's
The hospital of St Bartholomew may have been founded in *c.* 1190 but the foundation was enlarged after 1217 by Henry of Sandwich, Warden of the Cinque Ports, who is usually known as the real founder. The hospital was governed from an early date by the mayor and jurats of Sandwich who visited it annually on the feast of St Bartholomew. It escaped dissolution and was refounded by Archbishop Parker in 1562 for twelve brothers and four sisters.

Of the original hospital buildings only a thirteenth-century chapel remains, surrounded on three sides by eighteenth- and nineteenth-century almshouses. The chapel consists of a nave and chancel to which was added, shortly after foundation, a large north chapel and a north aisle which does not extend the full length of the nave. Under the arcade, between the chancel and chapel, lies a moulded effigy of Henry of Sandwich.

Sandwich: St Thomas
The hospital of St Thomas was founded *c*. 1392 by Thomas Ellis, a draper of the town, for twelve poor persons.

Before the hospital was rebuilt in the mid nineteenth century, it consisted of a building divided by a central passage; on the south was the hall, open to the roof, beyond which were the women's apartments. The men's dwellings were on the north side. Now only the entrance arch of the gateway remains and the stonework of a chapel window has been re-erected in the churchyard of St Peter's.

Strood: St Mary's
The hospital of St Mary at Strood was founded by Gilbert de Glanville, Bishop of Rochester 1192-3. It was endowed for a master, two priests, two deacons and two subdeacons. The hospital suffered losses during Simon de Montfort's attack on Rochester in 1264, and further declined in the fourteenth century when the hospital was exempt from taxation on account of its poverty. In 1330 a new, stricter set of ordinances was made as a result of a visitation finding neglect by the masters. The number of brethren was reduced to four but the situation did not improve, for in 1402 and 1443 the bishop took the administration into his own hands on account of the neglect of the master and dilapidations to the buildings. The hospital surrendered to the Crown in 1549 and was granted to the dean and chapter of the cathedral.

The last remaining portion of St Mary's Hospital was removed in the mid nineteenth century but excavation has revealed some idea of the plan and history of the buildings. The original hospital probably consisted of chapel and long, narrow hall with its long axis at right angles to the chapel, joined by a connecting archway. The hall was divided by a cross-wall, possibly to divide the sexes as at Lanfranc's foundations at Canterbury and Harbledown. At some time in the late fourteenth century the chapel probably collapsed, for it was completely rebuilt on the same plan. At a slightly later date, the hall would seem to have been converted into an antechamber by the insertion of a wall which cut off both ends, demolishing the central dividing wall, blocking the two entrances and making a new entrance possible with a porch.

Sutton-at-Hone: Almshouses
The almshouses at Sutton-at-Hone were founded in 1596 by Katherine Wrott, native of the parish, for four single poor of the parish.

The almshouses consist of four red brick, two-storeyed tenements under one roof, each with an upper and lower chamber and chimney. The almspeople also have separate gardens and a common hall.

Sutton Valence: Almshouses

The almshouses at Sutton Valence were founded shortly before 1574 by William Lambe, a London clothworker and native of the parish, to support twelve poor aged persons. The foundation was placed under the management of the Clothworkers Company.

The almshouses form a simple, one-storeyed row of six tenements with small gardens attached.

LANCASHIRE

Lathom: The bedehouse

The hospital at Lathom was founded *c.* 1500 by Thomas Stanley, second Earl of Derby. His foundation was intended for a chaplain and eight bedesmen. A chapel was consecrated there in 1509 providing a chantry to say masses for the soul of the founder.

An early-sixteenth-century, plain rectangular chapel forms the north-east angle of a group of buildings, including a row of almhouses, consisting of six tenements and a school. The complex is situated in the grounds of Lathom House.

LEICESTERSHIRE

Bottesford: Duke's almshouses

The Duke almshouses were begun before 1612 by Elizabeth, Countess of Rutland. Her son, Roger, fifth Earl of Rutland, traveller and soldier, endowed the foundation and directed that his heirs should complete it. The establishment was intended originally for the relief of six poor persons. The endowments have been augmented by successive earls of Rutland and the numbers increased.

The two-storeyed building built of brick and stone has been considerably remodelled. It originally contained fourteen bedrooms each with pantry attached. There was also a common room and kitchen. The entrance door is six-panelled with a three-panel fanlight under a seventeenth-century moulded stone cornice.

Leicester: The Newarke (Trinity) Hospital

The Newarke or Trinity Hospital was founded in 1330, possibly on the site of an earlier hospital, by Henry, third Earl of Lancaster. It was originally dedicated to the Annunciation of the Virgin Mary and was intended for a warden, four chaplains, fifty poor and infirm with five women to care for them. Twenty of the poor folk were to be permanent inmates, accommodated in a house next to the church, the remaining thirty were to be temporary inmates, housed in the infirmary hall. The foundation was greatly enlarged by Henry's son, enabling 100 poor, with 10 women attendants, to be maintained. In 1335, permission was obtained to transfer the hospital into a college called the Newarke.

The college was dissolved in 1547, but the hospital continued under royal patronage until 1610, when the Earl of Huntingdon, who had obtained the patent, sold it to the corporation of Leicester. The hospital was refounded by James I in 1614 and incorporated, with the mayor as master and dedicated to the Holy and Undivided Trinity. New statutes were promulgated limiting the number of inmates to 110.

Of the original hospital buildings, the dwellings of the permanent residents have disappeared, but a late-fourteenth-century chapel survives in part. The chapel was situated at the east end of the infirmary hall; the line of nave and aisle of the hall can still be traced, and in the entrance hall, part of the arcade is complete. The hall was originally seventeen bays long and consisted of nave and side aisles. At some time it was horizontally divided, cutting right across the nave and chapel. External chimney-stacks are shown in old views of the building.

Lyddington: Jesus Hospital

Jesus Hospital was originally built as a palace for the bishops of Lincoln. After the Reformation, the manor was granted to William Cecil, Lord Burghley, whose son Thomas, first Earl of Exeter, converted it into a hospital in 1602. The foundation was intended for a warden, twelve poor men and two women. The inmates were to be selected from honest workmen, artisans of handicraft, labourers in husbandry or servants who were unable to earn their living due to sickness, age or other infirmity.

The hospital stands north of the church adjoining the churchyard, separated from it by a stone wall. The existing building was erected by Bishop Russell (1480-95). The hall and great chamber stood on the first floor and were originally open to the roof. A flat wooden ceiling was inserted in the early sixteenth century. The hall was reached by a stone staircase at the rear and a timbered cloistered walk on this side was erected to enable the hospital inmates to reach the hall staircase. Under this covered way were the entrances to the fourteen inmates' dwellings which were converted from the kitchen and offices of the palace. There is a kitchen and scullery for common use and a garden with adjacent orchard.

Melton Mowbray: Maison Dieu

The Maison Dieu at Melton Mowbray was endowed and built by Robert Hudson shortly before his death in 1640. It was intended for the relief of six poor men aged fifty or more, of the town of Melton.

The almshouses are situated immediately east of the church of St John.

They are built of stone and are of one storey except for the three symmetrically placed gables. A four-centre headed doorway lies below the central gable.

Oakham: St John the Evangelist and St Anne

The hospital of St John the Evangelist and St Anne was founded in 1398 by William Dalby. The foundation was intended to maintain twelve poor men with a warden and chaplain. The hospital was not dissolved but, by the reign of Elizabeth I, only supported five poor, a warden and a sub-warden. Elizabeth refounded the hospital.

Of the original hospital buildings only a plain rectangular Perpendicular chapel remains.

Uppingham: Christ's Hospital

Christ's Hospital at Uppingham was founded in 1584 by Robert Johnson, Archdeacon of Leicester. The foundation was intended for fourteen poor men and one woman who was to wash clothes.

The hospital is situated a short way from the school close to the churchyard. However, the buildings have been much altered.

LINCOLNSHIRE

Lincoln: St Giles

St Giles Hospital was originally founded in the thirteenth century and intended for the reception of the poor. In the fourteenth century Gilbert d'Umfraville increased the endowment so that poor ministers and servants of the cathedral, who were past work, might be admitted in preference to other applicants. The foundation was not dissolved and in 1564 there were five poor men maintained in the hospital with the dean and chapter as patrons.

The only surviving remains are in St Giles church: a reconstructed twelfth-century doorway and arch leading to a side chapel.

Stamford: Browne's Hospital

Browne's Hospital, also known as All Saints, was founded shortly before 1485 by William Browne. The foundation was intended for the support of two priests and twelve poor persons. The hospital escaped dissolution but complaints were made against it in the early seventeenth century, probably to obtain the lands. However, James I supported the hospital and refounded it as a corporate body, increasing its privileges and immunities.

With the exception of the main building facing the street, all the other buildings beyond it — a small courtyard with cloister on the west, domestic rooms on the north and warden's lodgings on the east — were demolished in 1870. The warden's lodgings communicated on the south with the chapel, which extended to the height of the whole building, through a squint in a first-floor room. The chapel was built *c.* 1475 but not consecrated until 1494 when it was dedicated to the Virgin Mary and All Saints. It contains some original stalls, finely carved seat ends and misericords, as well as some fifteenth-century stained glass.

An elaborate carved oak screen separated the chapel from the inmates' dwellings on the ground floor of the infirmary hall. The inmates occupied a series of small cubicles (now removed), five either side of a wide corridor. At the west end of the corridor was a four-light window with two shields depicting the arms of the founder's family and the Browne crest. An entrance door on the north-west leads to a stone staircase which gives access to the upper floor in which was the audit room, muniment room and upper part of the chapel. The audit room, a spacious apartment, is still mostly original and contains some fine examples of fifteenth-century glass and a seventeenth-century fireplace on the north wall. The timbered roof extends over the whole range of the building. The entrance to the hospital at the west end of the main building was once a handsome gateway but was rebuilt in 1813 with considerable modification.

Stamford: Burghley almshouses

The Burghley almshouses were founded *c.* 1579 by William Cecil for a warden and twelve poor men.

The almshouses were built on the site of the hospital of St John the Baptist and St Thomas the Martyr, founded *c.* 1170. A few fragments of Norman masonry may be seen on the east corner of the main range facing the river. The main range consists of a row of two-storeyed stone almshouses with provision for ten rooms in the west range and two rooms in a smaller east wing. Access to the rooms was by a long corridor to the south and the upper storey is approached by a common staircase. Externally, the west range has five steep dormers to the river and six tall chimneys.

LONDON

Elsing Spital

Elsing Spital was founded by William Elsing, a mercer of London, in 1331. The foundation was intended for blind, paralysed priests and any space remaining was to be taken up by beggars who wandered about the city. By 1340 the house was administered by Augustinian canons but by the early fifteenth century the hospital was in debt and was suppressed in 1536.

Of the original hospital building only part of a fourteenth-century church tower remains.

The Savoy

The Savoy Hospital, dedicated to the Blessed Jesus, the Virgin Mary and St John the Baptist, was begun by Henry VII who left 10,000 marks in his will for the completion of his foundation which was intended to provide 100 beds. The hospital was only intended to provide lodgings for one night, except for the sick. Each evening, the hospitaller and matrons stood at the door to receive the poor who proceeded first to the chapel to pray for the founder, and then to the dormitory. The first master, a considerable pluralist, was accused of neglecting the statutes, and in his time the number of sisters fell from thirteen to seven. A master and four chaplains surrendered the hospital to Edward VI who appointed parts of its revenues and beds to his new hospital of Bridewell and Christchurch. The foundation was reconstituted and partially re-endowed by Queen Mary in 1556, but its former lands were never returned and from this date the hospital was in constant financial difficulties. In the reign of Elizabeth, the master, Thomas Thurland, was convicted of corruption and embezzlement of the hospital estates, and successive masters and chaplains managed to appropriate the revenues and the original purposes of the foundation were disregarded. Troops were billeted in the hospital during the rising of the Earl of Essex, and in the first half of the seventeenth century chambers in the hospital were let to noblemen and gentlemen. The foundation was finally dissolved in 1702.

The hospital was cruciform in design, a plan unique to England, but probably derived from the hospital of Santa Maria Nuova, founded in 1334 in Florence. The 'nave' of the hospital consisted of twelve bays and was *c.* 60 m long; the 'chancel' was 24.4 m long and the transepts measured *c.* 60 m overall. At the ends of both transepts there were large seven-light windows and externally the bays were marked by prominent buttresses. Over the crossing of the nave and transepts there was an octagonal glazed lantern.

This cruciform structure formed the dormitories, with every bed within sight of an altar: the eastern arm contained the Lady Chapel and the northern end of the north transept formed St Katherine's chapel. The internal arrangements of the dormitories are not clear, but they were probably divided into individual cubicles forming the 100 beds for the poor men. The smaller transept, on the north side, probably housed the poor men's hall, referred to in the building accounts, with three floors and a staircase on the east. The other of the smaller transepts contained the sisters' hall of two floors, with a set of seven chambers on the upper. Adjoining this hall lay the kitchen for use of the sisters. A block of chambers connected the great dormitory with the principal chapel of St John. This chapel is the only part of the hospital now remaining, and only the core of the walls is original. It consisted of an aisleless rectangle, the chancel being to the north, with an ornate ceiling and fine panelled walls. North-west of St John's chapel stood the main entrance gateway to the Strand, incorporating part of the old palace of John of Gaunt. To the south of the gateway stood a tower of two storeys which housed the treasury and exchequer rooms; over the doorway was carved the arms of

Henry VII. Further south were the master's lodgings and domestic ranges which lay alongside the waterfront. Other buildings, which also lay on the river front, were probably the lodgings of the Abbot of Furness and those of the Bishop of Durham's steward. These may have been older than other hospital buildings.

Walthamstow: Monoux almshouses
The almshouses at Walthamstow were founded in 1529 by Sir George Monoux, Lord Mayor of London, for thirteen almspeople, eight respectable poor men and five honest widows.

The buildings are situated on the north side of the churchyard. They consist of a two-storeyed range with the upper storey used as the school and lodgings of the schoolmaster. Only the west wall and gable of the existing building is original. It has a projecting chimney-stack on the end wall with four windows on either side.

Westminster: Henry VII almshouses
The almshouses at Westminster were founded before 1509 by Henry VII for thirteen poor men, one of whom was to be a priest.

The hospital was situated within the precincts of the monastery of Westminster. A detailed ground plan has been preserved, showing a two-storeyed range with six sets of two rooms on each floor. On the ground floor, at least, each chamber had its own privy overhanging the Long Ditch; this feature, and the plan of the almshouse, suggest that they may have been modelled on the lodgings built by Cardinal Beaufort at St Cross Hospital, Winchester.

MIDDLESEX

Friern Barnet: Campe's almshouses
The Friern Barnet almshouses were founded by Laurence Campe, a London draper, in 1612 for the support of twelve almsmen.

The almshouses form a long retangular brick building originally consisting of six tenements of two storeys with a later tenement added on the south-east. They have four-centred tops to the doors and low mullioned windows of three lights on the ground floor and two lights in the upper floor.

Harefield: The almshouses
The almshouses at Harefield were founded by Alice, Countess of Derby (died 1636). The foundation was endowed to support six poor women.

The almshouses stand 274.3 m north-west of the church. They are built of brick and comprise two two-storeyed groups of four tenements, separated by a central passage, so forming an H-plan. Over the passage, on the west front, is a stone carving of the arms of the foundress. The houses have gabled, tiled roofs with groups of diagonal chimney-stacks.

NORFOLK

Castle Rising: Trinity Hospital

The Trinity Hospital was founded *c.* 1609 by Henry Howard, Earl of Northampton, for the total support of twelve poor women presided over by a governess.

The hospital stands as originally planned and built between 1609 and 1615. It is constructed of Norfolk brick and is quadrangular in plan and one-storeyed except for the entrance gateway in the west range. The common hall is in the east range. The buildings were originally thatched but were reroofed in tiles in 1627.

Norwich: St Giles

The hospital of St Giles, also known as the Great Hospital or St Helen's Hospital, was founded in 1249 on the site of the parish church of St Helen to care for the sick. A meal was to be provided every day at the entrance of the hospital for thirteen poor men. Seven poor scholars were also to receive board and thirty beds were maintained for the infirm poor. Also entitled to suitable board or lodgings in an 'honorable' part of the house were all poor chaplains of the diocese of Norwich.

Up to 1547, patronage and the right to appoint the master were in the hands of the see of Norwich which seems to have consistently well administered the establishment throughout its history. In 1547, Edward VI granted the hospital to the mayor and corporation and declared the hospital church to be parochial. The establishment was then to provide for the total support of forty poor persons and maintain a grammar school and by 1645 there were beds for fifty-seven persons.

St Giles is a good example of a hospital built to an infirmary-hall type of plan with domestic buildings surrounding a cloister. The church has an unusual addition of porch and south transept, which include thirteenth-century stonework probably dating to its foundation, thereby affording a place of worship to local parishioners in place of their lost church. There is more thirteenth-century work in the groined roof of the kitchen of the master's house, but there are no other remains dating to the original hospital. A grant was made in 1375 for the building of a tower which adjoins the south-west corner of the infirmary hall. The chancel, with its splendid east window and fine panelled wagon roof, was rebuilt *c.* 1370-80; the infirmary hall and nave of the church were rebuilt in the time of Bishop Lyhart *c.* 1450-80. After the refoundation of Edward VI, the hall and chancel were divided horizontally to form more wards and were separated from the nave. At the same time a chimney was built inside the chancel and a chamber inserted over the Lady Chapel.

The cloisters and chapter house were also built by Bishop Lyhart *c.* 1450, although nothing now remains of the east range nor of the master's lodge, reputed to have been rebuilt by Lyhart and which extended eastward beyond the chapter house. On the north side of the cloisters was the dormitory (now the kitchen and bedrooms of the master's house). The refectory completed the quadrangle to the west.

Norwich: St Mary Magdalen

The hospital of St Mary Magdalen was founded *c.* 1119 by Bishop Herbert de Lozinga for the reception of lepers. Little is known of its history until it was united with the hospital of St Giles in 1506. However, the two institutions separated shortly afterwards, with different masters being appointed by the Bishop of Norwich. The foundation was dissolved in 1547.

The hospital was situated nearly 1.6 km outside the north-east gate of the city. The chapel has been restored and converted into a public library but it retains good examples of early Norman architecture.

NORTHAMPTONSHIRE

Brackley: The almshouses

The almshouses at Brackley were founded in 1633 by the will of Sir Thomas Crewe, one time Speaker of the House of Commons. His foundation was intended for six poor people of the parish.

The almshouses comprise a one-storeyed building with dormers built of stone and separated from the road by a low wall.

Brackley: St James and St John

The hospital of St James and St John was founded *c.* 1150 for the poor. In the fourteenth century the hospital received and maintained soldiers maimed in the king's service. By 1423 it was reported that the hospital supported no inmates and the revenues of the house had been grossly misused. By 1425 the hospital was refounded with a new constitution. In 1484, the patron, Lord Lovell, granted the hospital to Bishop William Waynflete who used it to form part of the endowment of his newly founded Magdalen College.

The chapel of the hospital still survives as the church of St James.

Higham Ferrers: The Bede House

The Bede House was founded, or possibly refounded, in 1423 by Henry Chichele, Archbishop of Canterbury, a native of Higham Ferrers. The hospital was intended for the support of twelve men and a woman, all of whom were to be aged at least fifty years. The foundation was not dissolved, and in the reign of Mary the mayor and corporation were granted the right to nominate the inmates.

The Bede house, situated in the churchyard, is a fine example of the smaller infirmary-hall and chapel plan of this date. There is some architectural evidence that it was rebuilt on the site of an earlier building, but the present one forms a rectangle, measuring just over 19.8 m by 7.0 m. The hall, of six bays, was originally subdivided into thirteen cubicles with a fireplace situated along the south wall. The hall retains its original oak roof and is separated from the chapel by a pointed arch. The chapel is raised about 0.9 m above the level of the hall and has a vaulted crypt below.

Externally, the building is of unusual construction, with alternate bands of different coloured stone. The west front has a large five-light window. There is a doorway in the north wall and two doorways in the south wall (now blocked) which originally led to the garden.

Northampton: St John the Baptist

The hospital of St John the Baptist was probably founded *c.* 1137 by Archdeacon William or Walter of Northampton, for the maintenance of infirm poor. Four altars were dedicated in the church in 1310, and chantries were founded therein in 1339 and 1340. In 1345 Bishop Buckingham issued strict injunctions for the regulation of the house, but these had evidently been disregarded by 1381 when a visitation found the inmates were ignoring the rules. A little before 1340, John Dalington, clerk, had made a grant of funds to the hospital to maintain eight poor people. Eight persons, three men and five women, were still being supported by this grant in 1535. The hospital escaped dissolution and was granted a new charter by Charles I in 1630.

The main hospital and chapel survived with a complicated, but interesting, architectural history. The main building forms a rectangle except for the east end which is slightly askew to conform with the line of the street. It is built of red sandstone and consists of two storeys. The upper storey contains the former brethren's apartments and extended the width of the building. A central passage on the ground floor divides the domestic apartments and hall from the inmates' apartments on the south. The hall was open to the roof on the north. This plan probably reflects a former infirmary hall with the separate dwellings now replacing the beds in the south aisle. The earliest extant part of the building is the west end, with the main hospital entrance dating to the fourteenth century and indicating possible rebuilding or alteration at that time. Some time after 1474 the hall was extended eastwards and a large fireplace built into the north wall of the kitchen in the sixteenth century. This fireplace was the only one in the building.

The eastward extension joined the main building on to the south-west corner of the chapel. The earliest datable architecture in the chapel is the east window, probably of the early fourteenth century, and may represent the only survival of the rebuilding of 1309. The west front is a particularly fine example of Perpendicular architecture. Late-sixteenth- or early-seventeenth-century work in the north and east walls may indicate that, at this date, the chapel was rebuilt to a narrower plan.

There were also many alterations in the sixteenth and seventeenth centuries in the master's house, which stood north-east of the main building and chapel until 1871.

Oundle: Lathom's almshouses
The Lathom almshouses were founded *c.* 1597 by Nicholas Lathom, rector of Barnwell St Andrew. The foundation was to support fifteen poor or lame women with a warden. The inmates were to be of good and honest conversation and none was to be a lunatic or have any infectious disease.

The almshouse buildings are two-storeyed with three gabled wings enclosing two small courtyards entered by stone gateways. The north court is original though much restored. The common hall was originally situated on the ground floor.

Rothwell: Jesus Hospital
Jesus Hospital was founded in 1591 by Owen Ragdale, a schoolmaster. It was intended for twenty-four poor, single men and a warden, all of whom should be aged at least forty years and have been resident in the parish of Rothwell for at least three years.

The hospital stands south-east of the church. The buildings enclose a small courtyard and are entered through a massive gateway of which only the arch is original. The main buildings form a long south range and two separate L-shaped wings. The northern wing was rebuilt in 1833. The sleeping cubicles were arranged around four common rooms, and a hall, situated on the first floor, contains a trapdoor leading down to a small chamber in which were placed any recalcitrant pensioners.

Weekley: Almshouses
The almshouses at Weekley were founded in 1611 by Sir Edward Montague for a master and six brethren with preference given to family servants.

The buildings (now a private house), standing south-west of the churchyard, form a two-storeyed range built of dressed stone. The façade has widely spaced mullioned windows, a four-centred doorhead in the centre with a gable over which has three obelisks and a large sundial. A frieze over the main entrance in an entablature corbelled out from the wall, bears the inscription: 'What thou doest do yt in fayth'.

NORTHUMBERLAND

Alnwick: St Leonard's
St Leonard's Hospital was founded by Eustace de Vesci, *c.* 1193, for the benefit of the soul of Malcolm, King of Scotland, on the spot where Malcolm was killed. After 1376 it came under the patronage of Alnwick Abbey. Little else is known of the hospital but it was in ruins by 1535.

Of the ruins only a few late-twelfth- and early-thirteenth-century fragments of the chapel still stand.

NORTH YORKSHIRE

Bedale: Christ's Hospital
Christ's Hospital was founded in 1608 by John Clapham, clerk of the
Chancery. His foundation was for a master, to be aged over forty and
literate as he was obliged to teach six boys, and six brethren aged around
sixty.

The almshouses, situated a short distance from Firby in the parish of
Bedale, were built in a garden of 0.4 ha. They now consist of a group of
six one-storeyed stone dwellings, with small mullioned windows, three
either side of a central chapel which has a large gabled and transomed
window. Behind the chapel lies the master's apartment.

Richmond: Bowes Hospital
The Bowes Hospital was founded by Eleanor Bowes *c.* 1618 for two poor
widows.

The almshouses were built within the former thirteenth-century anchorite
chapel of St Edmund. Much work of that date remains but the west wall
was rebuilt probably at the time of Eleanor Bowes' foundation.

Ripon: St Anne's
The hospital of St Anne at Ripon was probably founded in the early
fourteenth century but the founder is unknown. It was intended for the
support of four men, four women and a chaplain, with places for two
travellers. It was not suppressed.

The ruins of an early-fifteenth-century chapel remain with an arch
which would have led through to the domestic quarters.

Ripon: St Mary Magdalen
The hospital of St Mary Magdalen was probably founded by Thurston,
Archbishop of York, in the early twelfth century. It was intended for use
by travellers, and for relief of the poor and leprous, under a master,
chaplain, brethren and sisters. In 1342 an inquisition found that all the
sisters had died and the hospital was empty. It was then reconstituted for
the support of all blind priests born within the liberty of Ripon and also
for lepers. Another inquisition of 1352 found that the hospital supported
only four chaplains. It was also found that the master had demolished a
building for the housing of lepers as none had used it for some time, and
with the timber had constructed a chamber inside the hospital. Shortly
after 1535 the hospital was combined with the hospital of St John the
Baptist and refounded as an almshouse.

The hospital buildings, except the chapel, were rebuilt in 1674. A chapel, mainly dating to the thirteenth century, remains. It also contains a reused Norman arch and a four-light Perpendicular window.

Well: St Michael

The hospital of St Michael was founded in 1342 by Ralph Nevill *'pro remissione pecatorum meorum'*. It was intended for twenty-four poor, sick or feeble persons governed by a master and two priests. In 1535 the number was reduced to fourteen, but after the Reformation the foundation was re-endowed by the Cecil family.

The hospital consists of a two-storeyed building containing apartments for eight men on the ground floor and for eight women above. Adjoining it to the west is a small rectangular chapel. The arms of Nevill and Cecil of Burghley are displayed on the hospital.

York: Ingram's almshouses

Ingram's almshouses at York were founded *c.* 1632 by Sir Arthur Ingram, a mercer, who having made his fortune in London, settled in York. His foundation was intended for ten poor widows.

The establishment, built of brick, consists of two low storeys of ten dwellings, five either side of a central four-storeyed tower. A twelfth-century arch from the Holy Trinity Michlegate, is set in the north-east face of the tower, and projecting from the back of the tower is a single-storeyed wing containing the chapel. Each wing has two projecting chimney-stacks and three doorways.

York: St Anthony's

The hospital of St Anthony was founded in 1446 as part of the newly established Gild of St Anthony which had been licensed to found a fraternity for a master, two keepers or wardens, brethren and sisters. It was intended to maintain seven poor men and a chaplain. By the beginning of the sixteenth century, St Anthony's Gild had fallen into decline. A complaint in 1509 alleged great mismanagement and the corporation impounded the books and keys. From this time, the corporation seems to have exercised a certain amount of control over the foundation which may have abandoned its eleemosynary function for in 1551 the lord mayor and corporation ordered that the lead roofs on the aisles of the hall be removed and replaced by tiles, with the lead being sold and the hall fitted up as a house for poor people or a hospital. In 1604, by Act of Parliament, management of the poor passed into the parish overseers and the hall seems to have fallen into decay and continued only as a refuge for a few aged and helpless poor. A generous bequest in 1621 provided for substantial improvements to the building, but in 1627 the gild was dissolved. The hall became a military hospital during the Civil War.

The west end of the present building, consisting of a first-floor chapel and hall with antechapel on the ground floor, dates from about the time of the consecration of the chapel in 1453. Later in the fifteenth century, rooms on the first floor were converted into aisles either side of the hall. Towards the end of the fifteenth century, the building was extended to the east with the addition of an aisled undercroft on the ground floor and an extension of the hall by six bays. Further alterations, including the provision of chimneys, were carried out in 1621. Subsequent uses of the building have entailed extensive rebuilding.

York: St Leonard's

The hospital of St Leonard, also known as St Peter's, at York may have been founded in the time of William I by the secular canons of the cathedral of York for the reception of poor people. In 1135, William II changed its site and enlarged the foundation. King Stephen erected a chapel in its precincts and changed the dedication to St Leonard. The new foundation consisted of a master, 13 brethren, 4 secular priests, 8 sisters, 30 choristers, 2 schoolmasters, 206 bedesmen and 6 servitors. In the fourteenth century the dwelling house was in disrepair and a series of visitations found serious irregularities which led to stricter regulations being laid down in 1364. But from 1370 the numbers of the infirm began to decline and the hospital was dissolved in 1540 with the revenues amounting to less than a third of those in 1280.

A few fragments remain of what was a very large establishment. The ruins date from the thirteenth century and consist of a long vaulted passage and undercroft above which possibly stood the infirmary hall and chapel.

NOTTINGHAMSHIRE

Newark: The Bedehouse

The Bedehouse was founded by William Phillipott, a merchant of Newark, and endowed by his will of 1556. The foundation was for five very aged men who were to be blind, lame or unable to work for a living.

The almshouses were enlarged in 1738 and 1783 but the two-storeyed, sixteenth-century part of the house built of brick can still be identified, although much restored. There is also a detached chapel.

OXFORDSHIRE

Burford: The Great Almshouses

The Great Almshouses were founded in 1457 on land granted by Richard, Earl of Warwick. Warwick is usually known as the founder but their true creator may have been Bishop Henry of Burford. They were intended for the support of eight poor persons.

The buildings consist of a rectangular two-storeyed block with a large central doorway and two smaller doorways. Over the main doorway there is a plaque inscribed 'These almshouses were founded by Richard, Earl of

Warwick in the year 1457'. It is considered possible that these almshouses were a part survival of an infirmary hall but internal remodelling in the early nineteenth century destroyed any evidence necessary to confirm this.

Chipping Norton: Cornish's almshouses
The Cornish almshouses were founded in 1640 by Henry Cornish for eight poor widows.

The almshouses are set back from the road and consist of eight houses under one roof with stone gables and tall chimneys. They bear the inscription 'The work and gift of Henry Cornish, gent 1640'.

Crowmarsh: St Mary Magdalen
Very little is known about the history of the hospital of St Mary Magdalen. It was in existence by 1142 when the Empress Matilda conveyed it a grant of land. Several other grants are recorded in the thirteenth century but there is no further record after 1269.

A small Norman church remains with a chancel, nave and wooden bellcote. A north transept was added *c.* 1200.

Ewelme: God's House
God's House, Ewelme, was founded in 1437 by William de la Pole, Earl and later Duke of Suffolk and his wife Alice. The foundation was for thirteen poor men and two priests, one of whom was to be the master and the other to be a teacher of grammar for boys. In 1617, the post of master was granted by James I to augment the stipend of the Regius Professor of Medicine.

The hospital adjoins the west end of the parish church. A south aisle, called St John the Baptist's chapel, was added to the chancel to accommodate the bedesmen. It is connected to the church by a passage either side of which are doors to enable processions to make a complete circuit of the church. A flight of steps leads from the church into the quadrangle around which are the inmates' dwellings. Each dwelling, as ordered by the founder, had a sitting room on the ground floor, a bedroom over and a chimney. A covered walkway extends in front of the dwellings all round the quadrangle. The western side of the quadrangle contained the audit and muniment rooms and former master's quarters; on the north and south sides are the kitchen and fruit gardens for the master and brethren. At the north-west corner of the hospital is an entrance porch, built almost entirely of brick. This may have been added at a later date, but one of the earliest examples of the use of brick in Oxfordshire may be seen in the herringbone infilling of the timbered walls of the quadrangle side of the dwellings; the external walls are of stone.

Mapledurham: The almshouses
The almshouses at Mapledurham were founded in 1613 by the will of

Charles Lister who bequeathed lands to Sir Richard Blount for the erection of a hospital for the poor.

The almshouses form a long, one-storeyed range of chequered brick, originally consisting of six rooms with a garden for each inmate.

Oxford: St Bartholomew's

St Bartholomew's Hospital was founded before 1129 by Henry I for twelve sick persons and a chaplain. After the resignation of William of Westbury in 1312, master for forty-three years, there were a succession of wardens who mismanaged the hospital. In 1316, the king made new regulations reducing the number of inmates to eight and ordering the admittance only of the infirm. In 1326, the wardenship was granted for life to the Provost of Oriel College and two years later, the hospital was granted to the college who continued to support the eight poor but also used it as a place where the sick of Oriel College might retire for a change of air. The hospital remained in the hands of the college until 1536 when a settlement was reached and it became a city almshouse.

The hospital chapel, a small, single-celled rectangular structure dating to the early fourteenth century, remains. It contains fifteenth-century windows and doors and at some time a roof of three bays was inserted below the fourteenth-century roof. Remains of the main hospital range stand north of the chapel but were rebuilt by Oriel College in 1649. St Bartholomew's farm, lying west of the chapel, also formed part of the complex; it is of two storeys, built of rubble with attics and cellars, dating from the sixteenth century.

Oxford: St John the Baptist

The hospital of St John the Baptist was probably founded in 1191-9 by Hugo de Malaunay who was one of the first benefactors. It consisted of brethren and sisters for the sustentation of the poor and probably to provide lodgings for travellers. It was refounded by Henry III in 1231 and rebuilt on a new site. Although the hospital held a considerable amount of property in the fourteenth century, it was frequently excused payment of subsidies on account of its poverty. In 1437, it was granted to William Waynflete for the foundation site of his college. Early in the reign of Henry VII the college converted the lower storey of the chapel into almshouses consisting of three separate chambers.

Part of this vaulted chapel chamber remains, as well as the magnificent kitchen, or more probably the refectory, now incorporated in Magdalen College. The hospital buildings probably covered the same area as Waynflete's college.

Studley-cum-Horton: Croke's almshouses

Croke's almshouses were founded in 1639 by Sir George Croke for the support of eight almspersons, four of each sex.

The almshouses form a row of four small brick cottages under a steeply pitched thatched roof.

Thame: The almshouses

The almshouses at Thame were originally founded *c.* 1447 by Richard Quatremain in connection with the Gild of St Christopher. The foundation was intended for the support of six poor men. Three bedesmen and three bedeswomen were being supported at the time of the dissolution of the gild in 1548. Lord Williams of Thame secured the continuation of the alms foundation promising, in 1550, to support six paupers.

Williams probably demolished the original Quatremain hospital before his death in 1559, and rebuilt his foundation on the same site. The almshouses consisted of a range of six two-roomed, two-storeyed cottages of half timber and brick set at a right angle to the street. The upper storey overhangs and is supported on carved brackets.

SHROPSHIRE

Clun: Trinity Hospital

Trinity Hospital was founded before 1607 by Henry Howard, Earl of Northampton, and was intended for twelve poor men and a warden who were to devote themselves to the services of God.

The one-storeyed dwellings built of local stone form three sides of a quadrangle, the fourth side completed by a wall. The hall is situated in the central range which has two end gables and a fine group of central dormers. The chapel lies at the end of the west range next to the wall.

Ludlow: St John the Baptist

The hospital of St John the Baptist was founded *c.* 1220 by the Ludlow burgesss, Peter Undergod, for the relief of the poor and infirm with a regular brethren following a religious rule. The rights of patronage came to be vested in the Lacy family and passed, with the manor, to the Mortimers in the early fourteenth century. By the early fifteenth century the hospital seems to have become a small college of priests whose main functions were to serve the chantries and maintain obits in the Mortimer chapels of Ludlow castle. Despite this, and losses suffered during the sack of Ludlow in 1459, the hospital flourished during the fifteenth century and was held in considerable esteem locally, playing a significant part in the affairs of the town. A fire destroyed stores and crops in 1515 and the hospital fell into decline during the mastership of John Howard (*c.* 1505-28). In 1547, the hospital's estates were granted by the Crown to the Earl of Warwick.

In St John's house, facing Ludford Bridge, stands the south-west corner of the hospital site incorporating a tall pointed arch belonging to the chapel — the only surviving fragment of the hospital.

Ludlow: St John the Evangelist

The hospital of St John the Evangelist was founded by John Hosier, a Ludlow draper. He acquired the site in 1462 and the almshouses were built by 1482. After his death in 1486, his executors conveyed lands to the Palmers' Gild as a permanent endowment for the foundation. Inmates were restricted to members of the gild and one of them was appointed bellman, whose duties included summoning all the inmates to prayer in the almshouse chapel twice daily. In 1552 the endowments were transferred to Ludlow corporation.

The almshouses, consisting of thirty-three separate chambers each with chimney, were situated close to the church of St Lawrence where the Palmers' Gild founded their chantry chapel. The almshouses were rebuilt in 1758, but the very fine chapel of the Palmers' Gild can still be seen in the chancel of the church of St Lawrence. Mostly dating to the fifteenth century, it was dedicated to St John, and was used by the almsfolk throughout their history.

Shrewsbury: St Giles

The hospital of St Giles was probably in existence by 1136 and was apparently intended for the relief of leprous persons. By the early sixteenth century the abbey of Shrewsbury was patron of the hospital and the abbey began leasing out the hospital some time before the Reformation. Despite its close association with the abbey the foundation escaped dissolution. In 1636 the hospital was re-endowed by Walter Wrottesley, Earl of Tankerville, whose family considered themselves masters of the hospital.

There are no domestic buildings of the hospital remaining but the church of St Giles (rebuilt 1860-3) incorporates substantial remains of the hospital church. The nave is still basically Norman and the north arcade and chantry chapel are partly of the fourteenth century.

SOMERSET

Broadway: The almshouses

The almshouses in Broadway were founded in 1558 by Alexander Every, a clothworker, for seven people.

The buildings of local sandstone form a substantial terrace set back from the road. They have mullioned windows and porches with stone surrounds and cambered door-heads. Four prominent chimneys project from a largely unaltered frontage.

Bruton: Sexey's Hospital

Sexey's Hospital was founded in 1638 by Hugh Sexey for the support of twelve aged persons and a master (61).

The hospital consists of two courts; three ranges of the west court are original. The entrance is on the north side and in this range is the hall

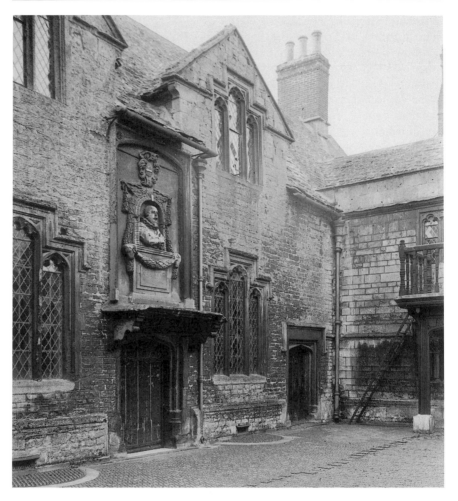

61   Detail from the façade of Sexey's Hospital, Bruton (1638).

with a storey above. The southern range contains the chapel which retains much of its original woodwork.

Donyatt: The almshouses

The almshouses in Donyatt were founded by John Dunster, a clothworker of London, *c.* 1624 and were intended for three poor men and three poor women.

The almshouses stand close to the church adjoining the entrance gateway to the churchyard. They form a two-storeyed range of six dwellings built of local sandstone. They have mullioned windows and four-centred door-heads. Each apartment has a bedroom and sitting room. Four prominent chimneys project from a tiled roof. A low stone wall and 1.8 m of garden separate the almshouses from the street.

Glastonbury: Abbot Bere's almshouses

Abbot Bere's, also known as St Patrick's, almshouses was a refoundation by Abbot Richard Bere, in 1512, of the hospital of St John the Baptist which had been in existence since 1246. It was intended for the support of ten poor women. The almshouses, like the hospital before them, were under the patronage of Glastonbury Abbey but were not suppressed with the abbey at the Reformation.

The hospital was situated just outside the abbey gates. The hall and domestic buildings have disappeared but the small sixteenth-century chapel remains as well as the entrance gateway. The gateway has a central carved panel depicting the arms of Henry VIII.

Glastonbury: St Mary Magdalene

The hospital of St Mary Magdalene was founded in the thirteenth century as an almshouse for men. Little is known of its history except that it survived the Reformation. After the Reformation it was known as the Royal Hospital.

The almshouses now consist of one row of cottages with a chapel at one end. The building was originally an infirmary hall and chapel under one roof. The hall was reconstructed in the fourteenth century and the chapel reroofed. In the sixteenth century it was converted into individual cottages of two storeys, destroying the hall roof and separately roofing the north and south aisles. In the twentieth century the row of dwellings on the south side were demolished.

Ilton: Wetstone's almshouses

Wetstone's almshouses were founded by John Wetstone, of Rodden, Dorset for nine almsfolk or families unable to maintain themselves through age or bodily infirmity.

The almshouses are separated from the road by almost 21.3 m of garden and a low-capped stone wall with central square entrance way bearing the following inscription: 'The howse was founded by John Wetstone, Gentlemen for the relief of the poor of Ilton in 1634'. The dwellings consist of a plain range, built in local stone, with two projecting wings and prominent chimneys.

Somerton: Hext almshouses

The Hext almshouses were founded in 1626 by Sir Edward Hext for almsmen who were to be aged fifty years or more and be chosen from certain named parishes.

The buildings present a fine stone façade to the street and comprise a single-storeyed range originally consisting of eight one-roomed dwellings. The doorways have cambered heads and are grouped in pairs with double niches for use as seats in the adjacent windows. Tall chimney-stacks project from the rear and there is a large garden still divided into equal parts for use of the inmates. The building was restored in 1967.

Taunton: Gray's

Gray's almshouses were founded by Robert Gray for ten poor women and six poor men. By his will (proved 1638), he settled £2,000 as an endowment for his foundation with the Company of Merchant Taylors as trustees to provide an annual allowance to the almspersons and a stipend for a reader who was to say prayers twice daily in the almshouse chapel. However, the Merchant Taylors declined to administer the trust and it was handed over to feoffees.

The almshouses form a two-storeyed range of brick consisting of sixteen tenements under one roof (**62**). The façade has two arched doors; over one is the coat of arms of the Merchant Taylors' Company and over the other, the arms of Robert Gray. Also on the front of the building in stone is the following inscription: 'Laus Deo. This charitable work is founded by Robert Graye of the Citie of London, esquier, borne in this towne, in the house adjoyning hereunto, who in his lifetime doth erect it for ten poore aged syngle women, and for their competent livelihood, and daylie prayers in the same, provided sufficient maintenance for the same, 1635.' For prayers, a small room furnished with pulpit and oak pews was used as an oratory. The women's apartments were on the upper floor, each provided with fireplace and pantry.

Taunton: St Margaret's

The hospital of St Margaret at Taunton was in existence as a leper hospital before 1174. Little is known of its early history. A legend records that it was burned down early in the reign of Henry VIII and rebuilt by

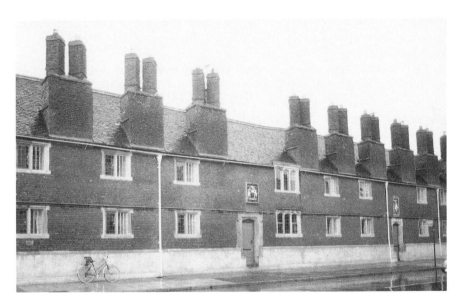

62 Gray's, Hospital, Taunton (1638)

Richard Bere, Abbot of Glastonbury (1493-1524). In 1547, the almshouses contained twenty-six inmates.

The architectural details of the simple row of stone cottages suggest that they were built in 1510-15 (**63**). The row consists of seven distinct tenements, each with a staircase leading to a room above. The end dwellings stand out from the centre five, but the roof is continuous, supported by oaken pillars which form a covered way in front of the tenements. In the front wall of the eastern house is a sculpted panel which displays the initials R.B. and above, a bishop's mitre, encrusted with sculpted gems. A house, standing at right angles to the westernmost tenement, but separated from it, incorporates the only surviving fragment of the hospital chapel.

Wells: St John the Baptist

The hospital of St John the Baptist was founded by Hugh de Wells, Archdeacon of Wells 1204-9 and Bishop of Lincoln 1209-33. The chantry-like nature of the foundation was probably responsible for its dissolution in 1539.

All that remains of the hospital buildings is a spiral stone staircase, incorporated into the priory.

Wells: St Saviour

The hospital of St Saviour was founded by Bishop Bubwith, Bishop of Bath and Wells, and built to directions left at his death in 1436. The foundation was endowed to support a priest and twenty-four poor men

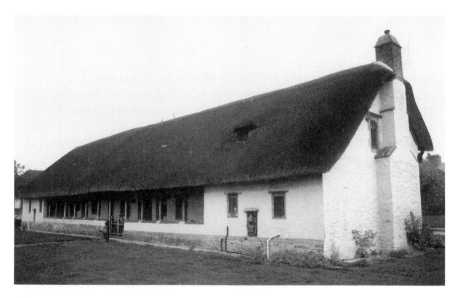

63 St Margaret's Hospital, Taunton (*c.* 1510).

and women. No lepers or anyone with contagious diseases were admitted and the more honourable places and beds were assigned to the reduced burgesses of Wells. In 1608, the almshouse was enlarged by a benefaction of John Still, Bishop of Bath and Wells, to provide relief for six more poor.

The almshouses (now much restored) are situated outside the north wall of St Cuthbert's churchyard. The chapel is entered from the street by a gabled porch and is separated from the hall by a carved oak screen. The hall, of two storeys, has a double row of rooms with central corridor on each floor. At the west end of the hall lies the gildhall, also provided by Bishop Bubwith. The wings lying to the south at right angles to the main range are the early-seventeenth-century additions of the Stills.

SOUTH YORKSHIRE

Bawtry: St Mary Magdalen

The exact foundation date of the hospital of St Mary Magdalen is unknown, but it was probably in existence by 1200. By the reign of Edward I the patronage was held by the Archbishop of York. It was intended for the support of certain poor persons under the rule of a master and warden. By 1405 the hospital, then seemingly reduced to the status of a chantry, was in the hands of Robert Morton, whose property was confiscated by the Crown. Despite its chantry-like nature, the hospital escaped dissolution, but in the later sixteenth century funds were misappropriated by the masters and it was not without considerable litigation that John Slack, appointed master in 1610, was able to obtain possession.

Slack's chapel was rebuilt in 1839. All that remains of the original hospital is a perpendicular image niche with a canopy, situated outside the chancel end of the chapel.

Tickhill: St Leonard's

The hospital of St Leonard at Tickhill was founded before 1225 but very little is known of its history. It is possibly identical with the Hospital in the Marsh, annexed soon after 1325 to the Benedictine abbey of Humberstone. It was dissolved in 1536.

The hall of the hospital has survived with a ground floor of ten bays and a fine timber-framed façade of 1470.

STAFFORDSHIRE

Lichfield: Dr Milley's Hospital

Dr Milley's Hospital was founded in 1424 on property given by Bishop Heyworth of Lichfield and Coventry to the sacrist of the cathedral and master of the Gild of St Mary for the support of the poor. At the beginning of the sixteenth century, it received a substantial endowment for the support of fifteen almswomen from Dr Thomas Milley, a canon residentiary of the cathedral, who probably also rebuilt the establishment between 1502 and 1504.

The present buildings probably date to Dr Milley's refoundation. They consist of a two-storeyed building of red brick which was originally L-shaped but reduced in size in 1906-7. The front range facing the street has mullioned windows and a central porch of stone leading to a wide entrance hall with the inmates' rooms on either side. The room above the porch, on the first floor, forms the east end of the chapel. The rear wing, extending back from the southern end of the front range, has a corridor on each floor which originally gave access to the almswomen's rooms.

Lichfield: St John the Baptist
The hospital of St John the Baptist was probably founded, or refounded, by Bishop Roger de Clinton *c*. 1140 for a prior, brethren, sisters and lay brethren living under a religious rule. An early-fourteenth-century visitation found the hospital had fallen into mismanagement and decay. Several reforms were ordered, but by the fifteenth century it had become a secular benefice with absentee or pluralist masters. In 1495-6 Bishop Smyth refounded the hospital to support 'thirteen honest poor men upon whom the inconveniences of old age and poverty, without any fault of their own, have fallen'. Bishop Smyth also drew up new statutes which decreed that the leprous and insane were not to be admitted and if any of the inmates became incurable, they were to leave the hospital. The hospital was also to serve as a school for a number of poor scholars. The hospital survived dissolution and continued to prosper.

The hospital was situated just outside the south gate of the city. Of the original hospital buildings, only parts of the chapel remain. The infirmary hall was connected to the west end of the chapel and would have occupied the north side of what is now the hospital quadrangle. On refoundation in 1495, it was enlarged into a fine house for the master. A new wing was added at right angles to the east end of the chapel, built of red brick, and was one of the earliest examples of the use of this material in Lichfield. Eight imposing chimney-stacks provided every apartment with its own fireplace. The buildings were much altered in 1720 and again in 1958.

Tamworth: St James
The hospital of St James was possibly founded before 1150 by Sir Robert Marmion. Around 1285 the master and brethren departed on account of their poverty. The foundation survived until it was dissolved in 1548 but was probably too poor to be serving any eleemosynary purpose.

The hospital remains consist only of the chapel (now restored) which had been converted into a dwelling. It consists of a small nave and chancel of Normal date (except for a remodelled west wall) with an Early English south doorway.

SUFFOLK

Bury St Edmunds: St Nicholas

The hospital of St Nicholas was founded by an abbot of Bury St Edmunds for a master, chaplain and brethren but the exact date of foundation is unknown. The first reference to it is in 1224 and by 1535 the chaplaincy of the chantry and mastership were combined. It was suppressed at the same time as the abbey in 1539.

The hospital stood a short distance outside the east gate of the town. There remains only the buttressed end of a building with the outline of a large window.

Bury St Edmunds: St Saviour

The hospital of St Saviour was founded by Abbot Samson *c.* 1184 for a warden, twelve chaplain priests, six clerks, twelve poor men and twelve poor women. However, in the time of Edward I (1272-1307) there were only seven chaplains and the poor women had been replaced by infirm priests. The hospital became involved in the quarrels between the town and the abbey resulting in much loss from rioters in 1327. In 1336 the hospital successfully resisted the imposition of a Crown corrodian but despite this, various corrodians were imposed throughout the fourteenth, fifteenth and sixteenth centuries. In 1528 the profits of the hospital were annexed to the abbey, being especially assigned for the exercise of hospitality at the abbot's table; the hospital was dissolved along with the abbey in 1539.

The hospital was situated outside the north gate of the town. It must have been a substantial building for Parliament met there in 1446. The site was excavated in 1887. Excavation revealed a long quadrangular building of the character of a hall with a 'gatehouse' at the western end. This is more likely the site of the chapel of St Thomas mentioned in 1386-7 rather than the site on the opposite side of the road commonly called 'Hospital'.

Dunwich: St James

St James Hospital was in existence as a leper foundation by 1189 and may have been founded by Walter de Riboff, one of its chief benefactors. The hospital was in difficulties throughout the fourteenth century. However, it survived the Reformation and, although greatly decayed in 1631, continued into the eighteenth century.

The remains of the hospital church stand in the churchyard of the modern parish church of St James and consist of a Norman chancel with apsidal east end.

Elmswell: The almshouses

The almshouses at Elmswell were founded by Sir Robert Gardener before

1619 for six poor widows. The almshouses comprise a single-storeyed terrace built of red brick with a steep central gable. There are five doorways and four groups of chimneys.

Eye: St Mary Magdalene
The hospital of St Mary Magdalene for lepers did not appear in the records until 1329 when Edward III granted the foundation the right to collect alms as they had nothing of their own to live on. Little else is known of its history but it continued in existence until the Dissolution.

The hospital was situated outside the town. Later buildings now occupy the site but contain reused material from the hospital.

Kersey: St Mary the Blessed Virgin and St Anthony
The hospital of St Mary the Blessed Virgin and St Anthony was founded *c.* 1218 but probably shortly after that date was granted to the Augustinian canons whence it became a priory.

Excavation has revealed the west range of the cloister of the priory to have been an early-thirteenth-century wooden hospital which was converted into the prior's house. The remains are now inside a farmhouse.

Little Thurlow: The almshouses
The almshouses at Little Thurlow were founded and erected during the lifetime of Sir Stephen Soame, a grocer who became Lord Mayor of London in 1598. His foundation was for the support of nine poor people, one of whom was to be able to read prayers daily.

The almshouses consist of three ranges surrounding a forecourt. They are of red brick and one-storeyed, except for a gabled centre; they contain eight apartments and a central room intended for the reader.

Long Melford: Trinity Hospital
Trinity Hospital was founded shortly before 1580 by Sir William Cordell, Speaker of the House of Commons and Master of the Rolls. The foundation was intended for the support of twelve poor men and a warden who was to be aged at least fifty. The inmates were to be a body corporate; in addition two honest widows were to care for them.

The hospital is quadrangular in plan with a courtyard facing towards the church. It is constructed of red brick and is seven bays wide, the first and last bays projecting as gable wings. The centre is embattled and has a cupola with windows of three lights below and two lights above. Three sides of the quadrangle consist of twelve separate lodgings for the almsmen, the fourth side contains the common hall, warden's apartments and accommodation for the two women. The building was much restored in 1847.

SURREY

Croydon: Whitgift's Hospital
Whitgift's Hospital was founded by Whitgift, Archbishop of Canterbury, and built between 1596 and 1599. It was intended for the maintenance of between twenty-eight and forty poor and infirm men and women. Preference was given to servants of the archiepiscopal see aged over fifty. The foundation attracted a number of benefactions in the early seventeenth century.

The buildings are of red brick and quadrangular in plan. The street frontage (western range) is symmetrical with three gables, of which the central one is taller and wider. In the centre of this range is the imposing entrance gateway which once housed the muniment room, and the external gable bears the initials I.W., the coat of arms of Whitgift and the see of Canterbury, and an archbishop's mitre. There is another gateway and entrance passage in the eastern range through which the garden is reached. This range also contains the hall and warden's apartments which were occupied by Whitgift himself on several occasions. The kitchen lies at the north end of the range with the chapel occupying the south-eastern corner of the quadrangle. The chapel is a small apartment but extends through the height of the two storeys; the original wainscoting survives round the lower part of the walls and there are also the original benches. The east window displays the arms of Whitgift and Canterbury. The almsperson's rooms occupy the remainder of the quadrangle and each room had a fireplace and deep cupboard.

Dulwich: Dulwich College
The Dulwich almshouses and college were founded by the actor Edward Alleyn in 1613 for a warden, four fellows, twelve almsfolk (six of each sex) and twelve poor scholars.

The almshouses have survived but were much remodelled in the eighteenth and nineteenth centuries. The college was arranged on a plan similar to that of Winchester College but smaller in scale and built in brick. The building formed three sides of a quadrangle with only an entrance gateway on the fourth side. The centre range contained the chapel and schoolhouse, while on each side were six almshouses. A tower was also erected but fell down in 1638.

Egham: Denham almshouses
The Denham almshouses were founded in 1624 by Sir Robert Denham, native of the parish and baron of the Exchequer, for five poor widows.

The almshouses comprise a simple single-storeyed terrace of five distinct, brick cottages under one roof. Each cottage has one room in front and a small back room.

Farncombe: Wyatt almshouses

The Wyatt almshouses were founded and endowed in 1618 by the will of Richard Wyatt, master of the Carpenters' Company of London. The foundation was to support ten poor men.

The buildings form a terrace of two-storeyed red-brick cottages under one roof with a central gabled chapel in which can be found a brass depicting the effigies of the founder, his wife and six children, an inscription and coat of arms. At the rear stand a row of imposing chimneys and inside the fireplaces are deep arched inglenooks with an oven on one side and window on the other.

Farnham: Windsor almshouses

The Windsor almshouses were founded in 1619 by Andrew Windsor of Bentley, Hampshire, for eight 'poor, honest, old and impotent persons'.

The almshouses consist of a two-storeyed row of eight brick dwellings, of two rooms each under one roof. The front is symmetrical with four plain gables and a central crow-stepped gable which has a stone panel inscribed: 'These almshouses were erected by Andrew Windsor Esq. in 1619 for the habitation and relief of eight poor honest old impotent persons.' A short flight of steps leads up from the street to each doorway and there is a central passage through to the small gardens behind. From the rear of the building project four massively built chimneys.

SUSSEX

Arundel: Holy Trinity or Christ's Hospital

Richard, fifth Earl of Arundel, began the founding of this hospital in connection with a college. When he was executed for treason, work was halted until his son obtained fresh letters patent and completed the scheme in 1396.

The foundation was for a master, who was also the chaplain, and twenty aged or infirm poor men. It continued to be supported by the earls of Arundel but was suppressed in 1546.

The buildings, once comprising a chapel, hall, master's lodging, brethren's lodgings and gatehouse, were probably set in a quadrangle, but all that now remains is a roofless rectangular building, apparently part of the western range.

Chichester: Cawley's almshouses

Cawley's almshouses were founded in 1626 by William Cawley for twelve decayed tradesmen of Chichester.

The buildings stand much as they were built in 1626 with some eighteenth-century additions. The almshouses are two storeys arranged in an E-shaped block constructed of Sussex brick. At the west end, either side of the entrance door, are two canopied benches which bear Cawley's initials and the date 1626. The chapel occupies the central block.

Chichester: St Mary's

Little is known of the early history of St Mary's but it was probably founded by William, Dean of Chichester in 1158. The hospital changed site some time after 1269 to the former quarters of the Friars Minor. The foundation suffered a decline in its fortunes in the late fourteenth and early fifteenth centuries when a commission inquired into mismanagement and dilapidation and by 1442 there were only two brethren and two sisters. It was refounded by Dean William Fleshmonger in 1528 and again refounded by Elizabeth I in 1563 as a corporate body.

The present hospital buildings constitute one of the most perfect examples of a medieval hospital in the country. It was probably built *c.* 1290-93 and consists of an aisled infirmary hall, originally two bays longer, and adjoining chapel. The hall is divided from the chapel by a rich screen dating to *c.* 1290.

East Grinstead: Sackville College

Sackville College was founded by Robert, second Earl of Dorset, in 1608 for twenty-one poor men and ten poor women, to be under the patronage of his heir. Building commenced in 1616 and was completed by Dorset's second son, Earl Edward. However, there were difficulties over the endowment since the Sackville lands were alienated by the third Earl of Dorset and the purchasers refused to accept responsibility for the college. Consequently the inmates did not receive their charter of incorporation until 1631.

The buildings comprise a spacious quadrangle built of sandstone. The façade is two-storeyed with three gables over the centre and end bays. The entrance doorway leads into the quadrangle. The opposite range has a small entrance to the hall and other apartments which were occupied by the members of the Dorset family. The hall contains a splendid hammer-beam roof and over the fireplace are the Dorset arms. The chapel and common hall are in the centre of the other two ranges. The whole, with its stone gables and chimney-stacks, forms a most attractive composition.

Lewes: St James

Very little is known about the hospital of St James at Lewes but it was probably founded by a member of the Warenne family soon after 1110 and attached to Lewes Priory. It provided for thirteen persons of either sex.

The hospital was situated next to the priory and probably consisted of an infirmary hall with double chapel. It was converted into a parish church in the fourteenth century and a row of twelfth-century columns, separating the nave from a later south aisle, remains in the church. A new hospital was built close by; this is probably represented by a chapel, now converted into a cottage, close to the priory gate.

Winchelsea: St John

The hospital of St John was founded *c.* 1292 and was probably the most important of the three hospitals at New Winchelsea. It was under the control of the mayor and commonalty but little is known of its history although it remained in use until *c.* 1586.

Of the hospital buildings, only the one gable of the range remains.

WARWICKSHIRE

Leamington Hastings: The almshouses

The almshouses at Leamington Hastings were founded in 1607 by the will of Humphrey Davis for the maintenance of eight poor persons of the parish in his house in Leamington Hastings which he had prepared for them. The charity was abused by other members of the family and an inquiry in 1633 removed any rights of the Davis family and vested the trust in six or more worthy knights and gentlemen of Leamington Hastings.

The almshouses stand a little to the south-east of the church. They form a long, rectangular building of two storeys, built of squared limestone, with thin alternate courses of red sandstone dressings. Over one of the doors on the south façade, facing the street, an inscription records that Humphrey Davis founded the almshouses in 1607 and bequeathed lands for their endowment which were detained for twenty-six years and only recovered in 'this present year 1633' with the help of Sir Thomas Trevor, baron of the Exchequer and lord of the manor. Internally they probably originally consisted of four apartments, but have been much altered.

Stoneleigh: Old Almshouses

The Old Almshouses were founded in 1579 by Dame Alice Leigh in the name of herself and her late husband Thomas who had been Lord Mayor of London. The foundation was intended for the habitation of five single men and five single women.

The buildings are situated just north of the church and consist of two groups of five two-storeyed spacious houses. Both ranges have symmetrical façades with five tall chimneys-stacks and each doorway opens into a passage formed by timber-framed partitions with plastered panels; a door either side gives access to the dwellings.

Stratford-on-Avon: Holy Cross

The hospital of the Holy Cross was probably founded *c.* 1269 by the Gild of the Holy Cross. It was intended for the support of poor priests and after that of other indigent persons. By 1389 the members of the gild were electing the warden and this probably indicated a change in the nature of the charity, since by 1442 the priests were no longer the recipients of the charity but its regular chaplains. The hospital was dissolved alongside the gild in 1547.

The almshouses stood opposite the gild chapel. The surviving buildings date to *c.* 1427 but were altered and enlarged from the sixteenth century. The original structure was of ten bays with an upper storey jettied on the front. The original entrance, a wide archway with cross passage, led to the rear courtyard. Chimneys were added in the sixteenth or seventeenth century.

Warwick: Leicester's Hospital

Leicester's Hospital was founded in 1571 by Robert Dudley, Earl of Leicester, taking over the premises of the combined gilds of Holy Trinity and St George. After the dissolution of the gild in 1546, the property was held by the burgesses of Warwick until 1571 when the buildings were given to Robert Dudley to found a hospital for a master and twelve brethren who, by preference for admission, should have been wounded in the wars, especially those who had been servants or tenants of the founder and his heirs. After the death of Dudley in 1590, his widow claimed the hospital's estates as dower, thereby putting the existence of the foundation in jeopardy until Lord Burghley intervened at the request of the master.

The hospital occupies the site and buildings of the amalgamated gild. The buildings are situated immediately inside the west gate of the city and include the chapel of St James, above the gate itself, probably rebuilt soon after 1383 when it was granted to the Gild of St George. The other buildings, including the gildhall, were rebuilt before the end of the fifteenth century, probably after the unification of the gilds. The buildings are set around a courtyard, entered by a gatehouse in the south range. The master's house, forming the north range, is much altered and may have been built or rebuilt after 1571. The north end of the west range is also incorporated into the master's house. This end of the range probably formed the service wing of the building which later came to be known as the banqueting hall. The range was two-storeyed at both ends with the central portion open to the roof. Much of the building was originally entirely timber-framed, carved with the devices of the Leicester and Warwick family.

Warwick: St Michael's

The hospital of St Michael was founded towards the end of the reign of Henry I by Roger, Earl of Warwick, for leprous persons, governed by a warden and brethren. The warden was a priest and served the chapel of the hospital which was granted to St Mary's College in 1123. It ceased to be used as such in 1367 and was probably rebuilt by the hospital in the fifteenth century. In 1545, there was no resident warden, although certain lepers were maintained there. The foundation was dissolved in 1547 but re-established with a resident warden by Philip and Mary in 1556.

The hospital stood outside the town wall to the north-west. The remains of the stone chapel, including the west gable-end, east end and early-fifteenth-century panelled wagon roof, are incorporated in an eighteenth-century cottage. Behind the cottage stands a two-storeyed half-timbered dwelling, probably the master's house.

WEST MIDLANDS

Coventry: Bond's Hospital

Bond's or Bablake's Hospital was founded in 1506 by the will of Thomas Bond, a wealthy draper and mayor of Coventry. It was intended for ten poor men, a woman and a secular priest. Thomas Bond's heirs evidently did not carry out his wishes, for in 1538 a suit commenced against his grandson to have the charity completed and the almspeople appointed. After the dissolution of the chantries the priest was replaced by a master and the chapel disused. The foundation continued to be well supported by the citizens in the seventeenth century.

The hospital formed two sides of a quadrangle also containing the collegiate church of St John and Bablake's Boys' Hospital. The two-storeyed north range of the hospital dates from the early sixteenth century but has been much restored. The central part of the range originally contained ten rooms for the almsmen with access along a corridor to the rear. The rooms were later subdivided. The apartments in the lower storey may have been in the form of cubicles, each with an individual window below a long clerestory above the partitions. At each end of the range were larger rooms on both floors (now altered); their use is uncertain but may have included accommodation for the priest and female attendant, the kitchen and perhaps the common hall. In the eighteenth century a chapel and chamber were mentioned as adjoining the hospital.

Coventry: Ford's Hospital

Ford's or Greyfriars' Hospital was founded in 1509 by the will of William Ford, draper, merchant of the staple and mayor of the city in 1497. Ford endowed an almshouse to be built for the support of five men and a women to care for them. Control of the hospital appears to have passed to the master of the Gild of Holy Trinity. The almshouses survived dissolution and in 1621 the lands were purchased by the city.

The street frontage of the almshouse is a splendid example of sixteenth-century timber construction. The two-storeyed front is symmetrical with a central doorway flanked by mullioned windows, while the jettied upper storey had three gabled oriels and richly carved bressumers, barge-boards and finials. The almshouses are entered from the street by a passage through the ground floor of the front range. This west range contained the nurse's quarters with the chapel above (now inmates' dwellings). The dwellings, formerly consisting each of a lower and upper room, were reached by an internal staircase (now altered) and led off a narrow courtyard. The room over the eastern range, through which a passage leads to the garden, is plainer in style and may have been added later when the number of inmates was increased. One of the upper rooms was originally the common hall and meeting place for the feoffees. The building was bombed in 1940 but has been well restored.

Coventry: St John the Baptist

The hospital of St John the Baptist was founded by Edmund, Archdeacon of Coventry, 1160-76, on land granted by the prior of the Benedictine monastery. It was intended for a warden and master, brothers and sisters, affording relief to wayfarers and the local poor. Little is known of the hospital's early history but in the fifteenth century the hospital was involved in legal disputes: in 1424 with the vicar of Trinity church over parochial rights, and more seriously, with the priory itself. An inquiry was held with the outcome in favour of the priory declaring the prior and convent were the true founders and patrons of the hospital. By 1534 the hospital was maintaining twenty beds for the poor but was dissolved in 1545.

The only surviving remains of the hospital represent the chapel, built of red standstone shortly before the mid fourteenth century. It originally consisted of an unaisled chancel, an aisled nave and north-west tower. The south aisle has disappeared and the nave is now 3.0 m shorter. Excavations have revealed remains from the first church on the site dating to the third quarter of the twelfth century but at a much lower level. The chapel may have occupied the north side of a quadrangle with the infirmary on the south side.

WEST YORKSHIRE

Kirkthorpe: Freeston's Hospital

Freeston's Hospital was founded in 1592 by John Freeston of Altofts for the support of seven poor, aged, unmarried men and one aged, honest unmarried women who was to be appointed as laundress and given the cottage adjoining the almshouse.

The almshouse is of an unusual design; square with central rectangular dining hall or common room, surrounded on three sides by seven apartments. The apartments are lower than the hall but their doors open on to it. There is a fireplace at one end of the hall which has mullioned windows in its upper or lantern storey. The laundress's or matron's cottage is adjoining.

WILTSHIRE

Chapel Plaster

Very little is known of this foundation. It was probably a chapel for pilgrims travelling to Glastonbury but it is not certain how it was originally used.

The chapel consists of nave and chancel, a west porch and north transept. The north transept probably formed part of the original hall built in the late fourteenth century which lay at right angles to the chapel with a large porch at the west end. The complex was two-storeyed. There was a major reconstruction *c.* 1500.

Devizes: Sexton's House

In 1615 the almshouse in Devizes, known as the Old Almshouse, was rebuilt in stone on a new site and new regulations were promulgated. When the building became the Sexton's House, after 1896, its four rooms were occupied by widows and two underground rooms were let to paupers.

The building stands west of the church and has mullioned windows and seventeenth-century dormers.

Malmesbury: St John the Baptist

The foundation date of the hospital of St John the Baptist is unknown but a document of 1389 records that the citizens of Malmesbury declared that it was founded by King Athelstan and they had the right to choose the chaplains. Little else is known of the hospital until it was confiscated in the reign of Elizabeth. It was purchased by John Stumpe, son of the famous clothier, Will Stumpe, who had purchased the abbey church. John Stumpe granted the house to the corporation in 1580 and by 1622 it was in existence as an almshouse.

Fragments of the hospital, including a walled-up archway and possible window, dating to the end of the twelfth or beginning of the thirteenth century, survive within the corporation almshouses built in 1694. It is possible that these almshouses occupy the original site of the hospital chapel.

Salisbury: St Nicholas

The hospital of St Nicholas was probably founded *c.* 1230 by Bishop Bingham who erected a new hospital near the site of an earlier foundation. The hospital suffered problems in the fifteenth century when on several occasions the foundation was exempt from taxation. In 1478 new statutes were laid down by Bishop Beauchamp, limiting the number of inmates to twelve brethren and sisters and a master. The hospital escaped dissolution largely due to a fight against concealers by the master, Geoffrey Bigge, and his patron, the Earl of Pembroke. In 1610, James I granted the hospital a new constitution, refounding it for six poor men, six poor women, a chaplain and a master.

In the thirteenth century there were two parallel buildings on the site; the northern building, probably of two storeys, may have been the earlier hospital which is mentioned in documents of 1227. The southern building was single-storeyed and consisted of a 'nave' of two aisles, separated by a central arcade of seven arches with a chapel attached to the east end of each aisle. The south chapel still stands and is a fine example of thirteenth-century architecture. Each aisle also had a west porch but only that of the south aisle remains. There was a major reconstruction of the hospital in 1498 when a considerable part of the building was demolished. At this time the master's rooms and former common hall were situated over the south aisle and the kitchen was south of the southern porch. The energetic Geoffrey Bigge, master 1593-1630, made further alterations. The hospital buildings were extensively restored between 1850 and 1884.

South Wraxall Hospital
The origins of the hospital at South Wraxall are obscure, but it may have been founded in the fourteenth century as a refuge for travellers.

The surviving remains date to the fourteenth century and consist of a chapel and hall which was extended in the seventeenth century.

Wilton: St John the Baptist
The hospital of St John the Baptist at Wilton was founded before 1195 for the reception of the poor. In the late fourteenth century there was a dispute over the wardenship when the hospital refused to accept the king's nominee, and by the late fifteenth century it had become customary for the senior burgess of the town to be elected prior. In 1535, there were apparently four inmates resident in the hospital but they had disappeared by 1548 when the master was accused of appropriating the income for himself. Nevertheless, the hospital continued in existence although the same charge was levied against the master in 1613.

One residential range of the hospital survives, consisting of four separate apartments under one roof. The range mainly dates to the early fourteenth century, but the interior reveals evidence of an earlier building, probably belonging to the foundation of the hospital. The chapel, probably remodelled at the same time as the dwellings, opens out of a passage running along the east wall of the residential range.

WORCESTERSHIRE

Chaddesley Corbett: Delabere almshouses
The Delabere almshouses were founded in 1637 by Margaret Delabere for five poor widows.

The five almshouses stand west of the church. An inscription in one of the end gables records that they were erected at the charge of Mrs Margaret Delabere for five poor widows in 1637.

Evesham: Bedehouses
The bedehouses at Evesham were built by Abbot Roger Zatton (1379-1418), probably in the early fifteenth century.

Just outside the precincts of the abbey, by the Norman gate, stands a fine timbered house which may be Zatton's bedehouses.

Worcester: The Commandery

The Commandery at Worcester, also known as St Wulfstan's, may have been founded by St Wulfstan before *c.* 1085. The original establishment was for a master, a chaplain and four poor brethren following the rule of St Augustine. By 1294, twenty-two persons were supported in an infirmary and three beds were provided 'in a decent place' therein for three indigent chaplains. The hospital suffered from poverty and mismanagement in the fourteenth and fifteenth centuries until Bishop Bourchier reorganized the institution in 1441. From that date the hospital probably thrived until 1524 when it came under the threat of suppression by Wolsey. However, Wolsey's death saved the foundation until 1539 when it was dissolved and became part of the endowment of Christ Church, Oxford.

The surviving building of the hospital, known as the Commandery, was sold to Thomas Wylde, clothier of Worcester, in 1545. Various surrounding buildings once formed part of the hospital, but the Commandery itself is an impressive timber-framed building of the late fifteenth century and was probably the hospital refectory.

NOTES

Chapter I Introduction

1. There is good surviving evidence of late medieval partitioning in the infirmaries at Monk Bretton and Fountains, as in the dormitories of Durham and Cleeve. For the most recent study of modifications in Cistercian practice, *see* Coldstream (1986).
2. Rebuilt superiors' lodgings of the late Middle Ages include Haughmond, and Croxden, Glastonbury, Castle Acre and Hailes, Neath, Valle Crucis and Whalley, Muchelney, Forde, Milton, St Osyth's, Much Wenlock, Cerne Abbas and Battle. For these and other 'amendements of lodging', *see* Platt (1984), in particular Chapter 6 'Bending the Rule'.
3. The literature on these changes is extensive and growing. Improvements in housing have been a principal theme of recent books by Colin Platt (1976, 1978, 1982, 1986). In addition, see the especially useful books and monographs by Mercer (1975), Smith (1975), Hall (1983), Brunskill (1985), Giles (1986, for the RCHM), and Howard (1987). Some of the more relevant articles might include Skipp (1970), Smith (1970), Alcock and Laithwaite (1973), Portman (1974) and Dyer (1986).

Chapter II The early hospitals c. 1200-1350

1. St Petronilla survived until 1539, St Nicholas had degenerated into a chantry chapel by 1534 but continued to function until 1539 (*VCH Suffolk* 2: 134).

Chapter III The infirmary-hall type c. 1350-1547

1. Grants are also recorded in: 1325 (*CClR 1323-27*: 421), 1328 (*CClR 1327-30*: 258), 1333, 1334, 1337 (*CClR 1333–37*: 13, 252, 640), 1340 (*CClR 1339-41*: 499), 1341 (*CClR 1341-43*: 185), 1344, 1345, (*CClR 1343-46*: 437, 619), 1347 (*CClR 1346-49*: 309).
2. Such tombs were probably common. The earliest surviving in the sample is in the chapel of the almshouse refounded by Abbot Bere in Glastonbury and most likely dates to its original foundation in the thirteenth century (Clay 1909: 172).

Chapter IV The late medieval hospital: The bedehouse

1. The triptych is probably Flemish in origin. It depicts the following miracles: the raising of Lazarus (centre), casting out of the devil from the dumb man with the restoration of sight to the blind man (inset right), the calling to life of the widow's son and the raising of the daughter of Jairus (inset left). The backs of the leaves display figures of St Paul, St James the Greater, St Thomas and St Peter (*Arch. Jnl* 1930-1; 429).
2. Archbishop Chichele also established a school at Higham Ferrers and contributed to the rebuilding of the parish church.

Chapter V Post-Reformation changes

1. W K Jordan estimates that 640 hospitals were established by 1480 and only a further 91 between 1480 and 1547, and of that total, 73 per cent were founded before 1350 (Jordan 1959: 257-8).

BIBLIOGRAPHY

CCh.R   *Calendar of Charter Rolls.* London
CCl.R   *Calendar of Close Rolls, 1272-1485.* London
CPL   *Calendar of Papal Letters.* London
CPR   *Calendar of Patent Rolls, 1216-1509.* London
L&P Henry VIII *Calendar of Letters and Papers, Foreign and Domestic Henry VIII*, J S
               Brewer, J Gardiner and R H Brodie (eds), London
PP   *Parliamentary Papers.* London
RCHM   *Royal Commission on Historical Monuments, England*, inventories in
               progress
SPDom.   *Calendar of State Papers (Domestic).* London
VCH   *Victoria Histories of the Counties of England*, in progress

Alcock, N W and M Laithwaite 1973 'Medieval houses in Devon and their modernisation.' *Med. Arch.* 17: 100-25
Arch. Jnl 1930-1 87
Arnold, A A 1905 'Cobham College.' *Arch. Cant.* 27: 64-109
Array Tipping, H 1924 *English Homes: Early Tudor, 1485-1558*
Ballard, A (ed) 1908 'The Chartulary of St Mary's hospital, Chichester.' *Sussex Arch. Coll.* 51: 37-64
Bannister, A T 1918-20 'The hospital of St Katherine at Ledbury.' *Trans. Woolhope Naturalists Field Club* 25: 63-70
Barker, W R 1889 'St Mark's or Mayor's chapel, Bristol.' *Proc. Clifton Antiquarian Club* 23-36
Bartleet, E S 1895-7 'The leper hospital of St Margaret and St Mary Magdalen, by Gloucester.' *Trans. Bristol and Gloucester Arch. Soc.* 20: 127-37
Baylis, H 1958 *Hospital of St John the Baptist without the Barrs of the City of Lichfield.*
Belfield, G 1982 'Cardinal Beaufort's almshouse of Noble Poverty at St Cross, Winchester.' *Proc. Hampshire Field Club and Arch. Soc.* 38: 103-11
Bellairs, Col 1892 'The Trinity hospital, the Newark.' *Trans. Leicestershire Architec. and Arch. Soc.* 7: 305-22
Bennett-Symons, F W 1925 'The hospital of St Giles, Norwich.' *Jnl Brit. Arch. Assoc.* new series, 5: 55-67
Bird, W H 1912 'Bond's and Ford's hospital Coventry.' *Trans. Birmingham and Midland Institute* 38: 1-7
Bowles, C E B 'Wirksworth grammar school and almshouse'. *Derbyshire Arch. Jnl* 16: 147-59
Boys, W 1792 *Collections for an History of Sandwich.*
Bradfer-Laurence, H L 1932 *Castle Rising.*
Brance, J 1971 'God's House, Southampton and its home farm in the reign of Richard II.' MA dissertation, University of Southampton
Brown, P 1981 *Buildings of Britain 1550-1750: South-West England.*
Brunskill, R W 1985 *Timber Building in Britain.*

Bullough, L 1961. 'A note on medical care in medieval English hospitals. *Bulletin of Historical Medicine* **35**: 74-7

Burden, E R 1925-9 'St Saviour's hospital, Bury St Edmunds'. *Suffolk Institute of Archaeology and Natural Hist.* **19**, pp. 256-85

Calendar of Liberate Rolls. London

Calendar of Memoranda Rolls. 1326-27. London

Carpenter Turner, B 1957 'St John's hospital and the commonalty of Winchester in the middle ages' *Proc. Hampshire Field Club and Arch. Soc.* **19**: 20-34

Carpenter Turner, B 1980 *Winchester.*

Carr, A M 1960 'The career of John de Campdene with specific reference to the hospital of St Cross, Winchester, 1383-1410.' Thesis, University of York

Cave, P 1970 *The History of the Hospital of St Cross.*

Chatwin, P 1952 'The hospital of Lord Leycester, formerly the hall and other buildings of the medieval gilds in Warwick.' *Trans. Proc. Birmingham Arch. Soc.* **70**: 37-48

Clapham, A W and W H Godfrey undated *Some Famous Buildings and their Story.*

Clay, R M 1909 *The Medieval Hospitals of England.*

Clayton, H 1984 *St John's Hospital, Lichfield.*

Cobbett, L and W M Palmer 'The hospitals of St John the Baptist and St Mary Magdalen at Ely.' *Proc. Cambridge Antiquarian Soc.* **36**: 58-108

Coldstream, N 1986 'Cistercian architecture from Beaulieu to the Dissolution.' *In* C Norton and D Park (eds) *Cistercian Art and Architecture in the British Isles* 139-59

Collier, Mrs 1897 'St Mary-le-Savoy and the old palace and hospital.' *Jnl Brit. Arch. Soc.* **3**: 220-31

Colvin, H M (ed) 1975 *The History of the Kings' Works*, Vol. III 1485-1660

Cook, A H 1925 *The Early History of Mapledurham.*

Cook, G H 1947 *Medieval Chantries and Chantry Chapels.*

Cooper, A T P undated *Sir Anthony Ashley's Alms House.*

Cranage, D S 1901 *Churches of Shropshire.*

Detsicas, A (ed) 1981 *Collectanea Historica, Essays in Memory of Stuart Rigold.*

Deverell, J 1879 *St John's Hospital and other Chantries in Winchester.*

Doe, G M 1900 'Some notes on the leper hospital which formerly existed at Taddiport, Little Torrington.' *Trans. Devon Assoc.* **32**: 289-95

Dollman, F J and I R Jobbins 1859-63 *An Analysis of Ancient and Domestic Architecture in Great Britain.* 2 vols

Drake C H 1914 'The hospital of St Mary of Ospringe, commonly called Maison Dieu.' *Arch. Cant.* **30**: 35-78

Dryden, H 1873-4 'Hospital dedicated to St John the Baptist at Northampton. *Reports and Papers Assoc. Architec. and Arch. Socs* **12**: 211-34

Dyer, C 1986 'English peasant buildings in the later middle ages (1200-1500).' *Med. Arch.* **30**: 19-45

Ellis, J 1946 'London alms-houses.' *Country Life* 22 Feb.: 346-7

Ellis, M H 1929 'The bridges of Gloucester and the hospital between the bridges. *Trans. Bristol and Gloucester Arch. Soc.* **51**: 169-210

Emmerson, R J 1884 'The hospital of St Bartholomew, Sandwich.' *Jnl Brit. Arch. Soc.* **40**: 56-60

Evans, K J 1969 'The Maison Dieu, Arundel.' *Sussex Arch. Coll.* **107**: 65-77

Fowler, J 1951 *Medieval Sherborne.*

Freeman, E A 1845 'On the architecture of the church and hospital of the Holy Cross.' *Proc. Arch. Institute* 3-18

Fretton, W G 1886 'The hospital of St John the Baptist, Coventry.' *Trans. Birmingham and Midland Institute* **13**: 32-50

Fullbrook-Legatt, L E W O 1946-8 'Medieval Gloucester.' *Trans. Bristol and Gloucester Arch. Soc.* **67**: 217-306

Fuller, A E 1883-4 Hospital of St John the Evangelist, Cirencester.' *Trans. Bristol and Gloucester Arch. Soc.* **8**:: 224-8

Fuller, A E 1892-3 'Cirencester Hospital.' *Trans. Bristol and Gloucester Arch. Soc.* **17**: 53-62

Gee, E A and **J S Purvis** 1953 *St Anthony's, York*.

Gibby, C W 1981 *Sherburn Hospital*.

Giles, C 1986 *Rural Houses of West Yorkshire 1400-1830*.

Godfrey, W H 1929 'Some medieval hospitals of East Kent.' *Arch. Jnl* **86**: 99-110

Godfrey, W H 1955 *The English Almshouse*.

Godfrey, W H 1959 'Medieval hospitals in Sussex.' *Sussex Arch. Coll.*, **97**: 130-6

Gottfried, R S 1986 *Doctors and Medicine in Medieval England*.

Gray, B K 1905 *A History of English Philanthropy*.

Hall, L J 1983 *The Rural Houses of North Avon and South Gloucestershire 1400-1720*.

Harris, R E 1970 'God's House, Southampton in the reign of Edward III.' MA dissertation, University of Southampton

Harrison, A C 1969 'Excavations on the site of St Mary's hospital, Strood. *Arch. Cant.* **84**: 139-60

Hayes, F J, D Williams and **P R Payne** 1982 'Report of an excavation in the grounds of St Bartholomew's chapel, Chatham.' *Arch. Cant.* **98**: 177-89

Heath, S 1910 *Old English Houses of Alms*.

Hobson, J M 1926 *Some Early and Later Houses of Pity*.

Howard, M 1987 *The Early Tudor Country House. Architecture and Politics 1490-1550*.

Hugo, T 1872 'The hospital of St Margaret, Taunton.' *Proc. Somerset Arch. Natural Hist. Soc.* **18**: 100-35

Humbert, L M 1868 *Memorials of the Hospital of St Cross*.

Humbert, L M 1888-9 'The hospital of St Cross, Winchester.' *Proc. Huguenot Soc. of London* 77-88

Hurst, H 1974 'Excavations at Gloucester, 1971-1973: Second interim report.' *Antiquaries Jnl* **54**: 8-52

Hussey, A 1909 'The hospitals of Kent.' *The Antiquary* Dec: 447-50

Hussey, A 1932 *Kent Chantries*. Kent Records, 7

Jordan, W K 1959 *Philanthropy in England, 1480-1660*.

Jordan, W K 1960a *The Charities of London, 1480-1660*. London

Jordan, W K 1960b 'The forming of the charitable institutions of the west of England.' *Trans. American Philosophical Soc.* new series, **50**, Part 8

Jordan, W K 1961a *The Charities of Rural England*. Aylesbury

Jordan, W K 1961b 'Social institutions in Kent, 1480-1660.' *Arch. Cant.* **75**: passim

Jordan, W K 1962 *The Social Institutions of Lancashire*.

Jupp, E B 1865 'Richard Wyatt and his almshouses.' *Surrey Arch. Coll.* **3**: 277-89

Kaye, J M (ed) 1976 *The Cartulary of God's House, Southampton*

Kerling, N J 1971-2 'The foundation of St Bartholomew's hospital in West Smithfield, London.' *Guildhall Miscellany* **4**: 22-148

Kerling, N J 1971-3 'The relations between St Bartholomew's hospital and the city of London, 1546-1948.' *Guildhall Miscellany* **4**: 14-21

Kershaw, S W 1824 'Whitgift's hospital, Croydon.' *Surrey Arch. Coll.* **9**: 353-64

Knowles, M D and **R N Hadcock** 1933 *Medieval Religious Houses: England and Wales*.

Knowles, M D and **R N Hadcock** 1957 'Additions and corrections to *Medieval Religious Houses: England and Wales*.' *English Hist. Review* **72**: 60-87

Kusaba, Y 1983 'The architectural history of the hospital of the church of St Cross, Winchester.' Ph.D thesis, University of Indiana

Latimer, J 1901. 'The hospital of St John, Bristol.' *Trans. Bristol and Gloucester Arch. Soc.* **24**: 172-8

Lee, S (ed) 1900 *Dictionary of National Biography*.

Leech, R H and **A D McWhirr** 1982 'Excavations at St John's hospital, Cirencester.'

Trans. Bristol and Gloucester Arch. Soc. **100**: 191-209

Lees, E undated 'History of the hospital of St Wulfstan, commonly called The Commandery, Worcester.' *Reports and Papers Assoc. Archit. and Arch. Soc.* **9** 135-40

Leighton, W 1913 'Trinity hospital (Bristol).' *Trans. Bristol and Gloucester Arch. Soc.* **36**: 251-87

Leonard, E M 1900 *The Early History of English Poor Relief.*

Little, F 1627 *A Monument of Christian Munificence* (ed. C D Cobhan 1872).

Livett, G M 1929-30 'Notes on the hospital of St Nicholas, Harbledown.' *Arch. Jnl* **86**: 294-8

Loftie, W J 1878 *Memorials of the Savoy.*

Luce, R H 1949-59 'The St John's almshouse, Malmesbury.' *Wiltshire Arch. Mag.* **53**: 118-26

Lynham, C 1906 'The chapel of the hospital of St James, Wigginton, Tamworth. *Jnl Brit. Arch. Assoc.* new series, **12**: 125-7

Lynham, C 1908 'The hospital of St James, Tamworth.' *Arch. Jnl* **65**: 61-3

McWhirr, A 1976 *Studies in the Archaeology and History of Cirencester.* British Arch. Reports, 30

Markham, C A 1897-8 'Hospital of St David or the Holy Trinity, Kingsthorpe, Northamptonshire.' *Reports and Papers of the Assoc. Architec. and Arch. Socs* **24**: 170-9

Mayo, C H 1893 'Report on the almshouse of St John the Baptist and St John the Evangelist.' *Proc. Dorset Natural Hist. Arch. Field Club* **14**: xiv-xxvii

Mayo, C H 1926 *Almshouse of St John the Baptist and St John the Evangelist, Sherborne.*

Meade, D N 1968 'The hospital of St Giles at Kepier, near Durham 1112-1545.' *Trans. Durham and Northumberland Arch. and Architect. Soc.* new series, **1**: 45-55

Med. Arch. 1968 **12**: 56

Mellows, W T 1917-18 'The medieval hospitals of Peterborough.' *Reports and Papers of the Assoc. Architec. and Arch. Socs* **34**: 281-308

Melville, Lord 1899 'Lathom hospital.' *Jnl Brit. Arch. Assoc.* second series, **5**: 29-34

Mercer, E 1975 *English Vernacular Houses.*

Messent, C J W 1934 *Monastic Remains in Norfolk and Suffolk.*

Moberley, the Reverend 1891 'St Nicholas hospital, Salisbury.' *Wiltshire Arch. Mag.* **25**: 119-64

Money, W 1875-6 'The history of the Maison Dieu or hospital of Sir Richard Abberbury at Donnington.' *Proc. Newbury and District Field Club* 55-62

Morgan, F C 1952 'The accounts of St Katherine's hospital, Ledbury 1584-1595.' *Trans. Woolhope Naturalists Field Club* **34**: 88-132

National Association of Almshouses Archives

Newman, J 1969a *The Buildings of England: North and East Kent.*

Newman, J 1969b *The Buildings of England: West Kent and the Weald.*

Newton, P A 1966 'William Browne's hospital at Stamford: a note on the early history and the date of the buildings.' *Antiquaries Jnl* **46**: 283-6

Norton, C and **D Park** (ed) 1986 *Cistercian Art and Architecture in the British Isles.*

Palmer, P G 1917 'Inventory of Abbot's Hospital, Guildford, 1633.' *Surrey Arch. Coll.* **30**: 38-53

Palmer, P G 1927 *The Statutes of the Hospital of the Blessed Trinity, Guildford, A.D. 1629.*

Parker, G 1922 'Early Bristol medical institutions, the medieval hospitals and barber surgeons.' *Trans. Bristol and Gloucester Arch. Soc.* **44**: 155-78

Parker, J 1866 *The Architectural Antiquities of the City of Wells.*

Parker, J 1885 'Account of the hospital of St John the Baptist, Wycombe. *Archaeologia* **48**: 285-92

Parker, J 1898a 'Wycombe and its antiquities.' *Records of Buckingham* **5**: 153-76

Parker, J 1898b 'The hospital of St John the Baptist, Wycombe.' *Records of Buckingham* **5**: 245-8

Parkin, E W 1970 'Cogan house, St Peter's, Canterbury.' *Arch. Cant.* **85**: 123-38

Parsons, J E 1968 'Archaeological observations at Kepier hospital, 1961. *Trans. Durham and Northumberland Antiq. and Arch. Soc.* new series, **1**: 59-71

Pears, S A 1966 'The Lord Leycester hospital, Warwick.' *Trans. Ancient Mon. Soc.* new series, **13**: 35-41

Pevsner, N 1951 *The Buildings of England.* Rev edn in progress

Platt, C 1976 *The English Medieval Town.*

Platt, C 1978 *Medieval England.*

Platt, C 1982 *The Castle in Medieval England and Wales.*

Platt, C 1984 *The Abbeys and Priories of Medieval England.*

Platt, C 1986 *Late Medieval and Renaissance Britain.*

Ponting, C E 1892 'Architectural notes on the places visited by the society in 1891: the hospital of St John the Baptist, Wilton.' *Wiltshire Arch. Mag.* **26**: 193-4

Portman, D 1974 'Vernacular building in the Oxford region in the sixteenth and seventeenth centuries.' *In* C W Chalklin and M A Havinden (eds) *Rural Change and Urban Growth 1500-1800*: 135-70

Power, d'Arcy, Sir 1923 *A Short History of St Bartholomew's Hospital, London, 1123-1923.*

Preston, A E 1929 *Christ's Hospital, Abingdon.*

Pritchard, J E 1911 'Notes on Trinity Hospital chapel and almshouses, Bristol.' *Trans. Bristol and Gloucester Arch. Soc.* **34**: 93

Ragg, F W 1909 'Charters to St Peter's (St Leonard's) hospital, York and Byland abbey.' *Trans. Cumberland and Westmorland Antiq. and Arch. Soc.* **9**: 236-70

Raines, F R (ed) 1862 *History of the Chantries in the County Palatine of Lancashire.*

Rawcliffe, C 1984 'The hospitals of later medieval London.' *Medical History* **28**: 1-21

Records of Buckingham 1906 **9**: 310-11

Rigold, S E 1964 'Two Kentish hospitals re-examined: St Mary, Ospringe and St Stephen and St Thomas, New Romney.' *Arch. Cant.* **79**: 31-69

Robson, H L 1953 'The medieval hospitals of Durham.' *Trans. Durham and Northumberland Antiq. and Arch. Soc.* **22**: 33-56

Robson, H L 1953 'The medieval hospitals of Durham.' *Sunderland Antiq. Soc.* **22**: 33-56

Roper, I M 1903 'Effigies of Bristol.' *Trans. Bristol and Gloucester Arch. Soc.* **26**: 214-87

Ross, C (ed) 1959 *Cartulary of St Mark's Hospital, Bristol.* Bristol Record Soc. Publications 21

Rushforth, G 1927 'The painted glass in the lord mayor's chapel, Bristol. *Trans. Bristol and Gloucester Arch. Soc.* **49**: 301-31

Salter, H E (ed) 1914-17 *Cartulary of the Hospital of St John the Baptist, Oxford.* 3 vols, Oxford

Salzman, L F 1967 *Building in England down to 1540. A Documentary History.* 2nd edn

Sampson, W A 1909 'The almshouses of Bristol.' *Trans. Bristol and Gloucester Arch. Soc.* **27**: 84-104

Sayle, C E 1898-1903 'The chapel of the hospital of St John, Duxford' (Whittlesford Bridge).' *Proc. Cambridgeshire Antiq. Soc.* **10**: 375-83

Seymour, M 1947 'The organisation, personnel and functions of the medieval hospital in the later Middle Ages.' Thesis University of London

Shiffner, G 1849 'On the hospital of St Mary in Chichester.' *Sussex Arch. Coll.* **2**: 1-6

Sieveking, W G undated 'God's hostels; two ancient English almshouses.' *Berkshire, Buckinghamshire, Oxfordshire Arch. Jnl* **12**: 80-1

Skillington, F E 1973-4 'The Trinity hospital, Leicester.' *Trans. Leicestershire Arch. and Hist. Soc.* **49**: 1-17

Skipp, V H T 1970 'Economic and social change in the Forest of Arden, 1530-1649.' *Agricultural History Review* **18**: 84-111

Smith, G H 1979 'The excavation of the hospital of St Mary, Ospringe, commonly called Maison Dieu.' *Arch. Cant.* **95**: 81-184

Smith, H P 1926 'The almshouses of St George in the town of Poole.' *Dorset Natural Hist. and Arch. Field Club* **47**: 155-8

Smith, J T 1970 'The evolution of the English peasant house to the late seventeenth century: the evidence of buildings.' *Jnl Brit. Arch. Assoc.* **33**: 122-47

Smith, P 1975 *Houses of the Welsh Countryside.*

Somerville, R 1960 *The Savoy.*

Spittle, D 1974 'Browne's hospital, Stamford.' *Arch. Jnl* **131**: 351-2

Spoor, the Reverend 1891 'The almshouse chapel, Hadleigh and the will of archdeacon Pykenham.' *Proc. Suffolk Institute of Arch. and Natural Hist.* **7**: 378-80

Statutes of the Realm. London

Stubbes, P 1595 *Anatomy of Abuses.*

Swainson, C A 1872 'The hospital of St Mary in Chichester.' *Sussex Arch. Coll.* **24**: 41-62

Taylor, J 1878-9 'The hospital of St Mark, commonly called Billeswick or Gaunt's hospital.' *Trans. Bristol and Gloucester Arch. Soc.* **3**: 241-58

Taylor, K C L 1946-8 'The civil government of Gloucester,' 1640-46. *Trans. Bristol and Gloucester Arch. Soc.* **67**: 59-118

Templeman, G (ed) 1944 *Records of the Holy Trinity, St Mary, St John the Baptist, St Katherine.*

Tester, P J 1964 'Notes on the medieval chantry college at Cobham.' *Arch. Cant.* **79**: 109-20

Thomas, V 1889 'Notes on St Margaret's chapel and hospital, Wimborne.' *Proc. Dorset Natural Hist. and Antiq. Field Club* **10**: xxvi-xxvii

Thompson, A H 1937 *The History of the Hospital and New College of the Annunciation of St Mary in the Newarke, Leicester.*

Tibbits, E G 1936 'The hospital of Robert, earl of Leicester, in Warwick.' *Trans. Birmingham Arch. Soc.* **60**: 112-44

Tierney, B 1959 *Medieval Poor Law.*

Tierney, M A 1834 *The History and Antiquities of the Castle and Town of Arundel.*

Trans. Bristol and Gloucester Arch. Soc. 1958 **74**: 180

Turner, T H and **J H Parker**, 1851-9 *Some Account of the Domestic Architecture in England from the Conquest to the Reign of Henry VIII.* 3 vols

Valor Ecclesiasticus, temp. Henrici VIII, auctoritate Regia Institutis 1810-34 (eds J Caley and J Hunter), Record Commission

Vowell, I 1947 *The Description of the City of Exeter.*

Walcott, M E C 1868 'Inventory of St Mary's hospital or Maison Dieu, Dover.' *Arch. Cant.* **7**: 272-80

Walcott, M E C 1870 'Notes on the inventories and valuation of religious houses at the time of the Dissolution, from the Public Record Office.' *Archaeologia* **43**: 210-49

Warren, W T 1889 *St Cross Hospital.*

Westlake, H F 1919 *The Parish Gilds of Medieval England.*

Wildman, W B 1902 *A Short History of Sherborne.*

Woodward, B B 1974 *A History and Description of Winchester.*

Wordsworth, C (ed) 1902 *The Fifteenth Century Cartulary of St Nicholas Hospital, Salisbury.*

Wright, H P 1873 *The Story of the Domus Dei of Portsmouth.*

Wright, H P 1885 *The Story of the Domus Dei of Chichester.*

Wright, H P 1890 *The Story of the Domus Dei of Stamford.*

INDEX